INTERMITTENT FASTING FOR WOMEN OVER 50

STEP BY STEP GUIDE TO ELEVATE ENERGY AND MOOD, INCLUDING SLEEP AND STRESS MANAGEMENT, SUSTAINABLE WEIGHT LOSS AND HEALTH IMPROVEMENT POST MENOPAUSE

C. GERVAIS

TABLE OF CONTENTS

INTRODUCTION

Let's start with a story. Meet Linda. She's 52, a mother of three, and recently retired. Linda has always been active, but after menopause, she noticed something strange. Despite her best efforts, the weight started to creep up. Her energy levels dipped, and her mood swung like an unpredictable pendulum. She felt like her body was betraying her. Does this sound familiar? If so, you're not alone. Many women over 50 experience these changes and feel lost in a sea of conflicting health advice.

Linda's story is not unique, but it is powerful. It highlights the very real struggles faced by women post-menopause. And that's why this book exists—to help you navigate these changes with confidence and ease.

I'm deeply passionate about helping women over 50 regain control over their health. My commitment to this cause is grounded in science-backed research and practical, evidence-based strategies. This book aims to empower you with knowledge and tools to boost your energy, elevate your mood, manage your weight, and improve your overall health after menopause.

So, what's the big idea here? Intermittent fasting. Unlike other books on the subject, this one is tailored specifically for women over 50. It addresses the hormonal and metabolic shifts that occur during menopause. We'll use charts and diagrams to make complex information simple and accessible.

Intermittent fasting is not just about skipping meals. It's a pattern of eating that cycles between periods of eating and fasting. There are various methods, like the 16/8 method, where you fast for 16 hours and eat during an 8-hour window. Another popular method is the 5:2, where you eat normally for five days and restrict calories for two. The beauty of intermittent fasting is its adaptability. You can personalize it to fit your lifestyle and needs.

Now, I know what you're thinking. "Is intermittent fasting safe for me?" "Will I be able to stick with it?" "Isn't it just another fad?" These are valid concerns. Many people are skeptical, especially women over 50, who have unique health needs. Throughout this book, I will address these misconceptions and debunk the myths with solid scientific evidence and real-life success stories.

The structure of this book is designed with clarity and precision, guiding you through every aspect of intermittent fasting with a well-defined plan. We begin by unraveling the concept of intermittent fasting and its numerous advantages. Progressing further, we will tailor a fasting regimen that aligns with your personal health goals and lifestyle. Key topics such as managing changes in metabolism post-menopause, achieving hormonal equilibrium, and formulating nutritional strategies will be thoroughly explored. To aid in your journey, you'll find practical advice, specific fasting schedules, and detailed meal plans to ensure a smooth and informed path forward. Embedded within each chapter is rigorous, science-based research, ensuring that every piece of advice has a foundation in proven studies, backed by expert insights from the fields of nutrition and gerontology. We aim to simplify the complexities of intermittent fasting through straightforward explanations, complemented by illustrative diagrams and charts, making the science digestible and engaging. But this book offers more than just weight loss strategies; it's a comprehensive guide to enhancing your overall well-being. Discover how intermittent fasting can boost your energy, elevate your mood, assist in stress management, and improve your sleep quality. Our objective is to support you in feeling your best, not just achieving a particular dress size. This book is specifically crafted with your unique needs in mind, addressing the hormonal and metabolic adjustments that accompany menopause. With the aid of diagrams and charts, we'll make the underpinning science accessible and straightforward. By adopting this method, you'll be able to maximize the benefits of intermittent fasting effectively. As you turn these pages, approach them with a dedication to self-care. Embrace patience and maintain consistency; the outcomes you seek will unfold in time, promising significant rewards. This journey is not just about following a guide—it's about transforming your health and vitality during the post-menopausal stage of your life. You are not merely reading; you are stepping into a life-altering adventure toward a healthier, more vibrant you. Welcome to this pivotal chapter in your life's story. Let's embark on this remarkable journey together. We'll start with understanding intermittent fasting and its benefits. From there, we'll dive into customizing a fasting plan that suits you. We'll cover managing post-menopausal metabolism, hormonal balance, and nutritional strategies. Practical tips, schedules, and meal plans will guide you every step of the way.

Expect to find science-backed research in every chapter. Each recommendation is grounded in studies and consultations with experts in nutrition and gerontology. We'll demystify intermittent fasting with clear explanations and easy-to-follow diagrams and charts.

This book is not just about weight loss. It's about holistic health improvement. We'll explore how intermittent fasting can elevate your energy levels, improve your mood, help manage stress, and enhance your sleep quality. The goal is to help you feel better overall, not just to fit into a smaller dress size.

Unlike other books, this one is tailored for you. It addresses the hormonal and metabolic shifts that occur during menopause. Charts and diagrams will make the science easy to understand. This approach ensures you get the most out of intermittent fasting.

I encourage you to keep an open mind. This book is designed with your specific needs in mind. Approach it with a commitment to self-care. Patience and consistency are key. The results will come, and they'll be worth it.

So, let's start this journey together. This book is your partner in reclaiming your vitality and joy in the post-menopausal phase of your life. You're not just reading a guide; you're embarking on a transformative journey toward a healthier, more vibrant version of yourself.

Welcome to your new chapter. Let's make it extraordinary.

1

UNDERSTANDING INTERMITTENT FASTING AND MENOPAUSE

R emember the time when you could eat a whole pizza and your metabolism would just laugh it off? Yeah, me neither. Post-menopause, our bodies seem to have their own agenda, and it's not always in line with our wishes. I bet you've noticed changes in your body that make you feel like you're living in someone else's skin. Weight gain, energy dips, mood swings—the whole package. It's like Mother Nature decided to throw a curve-ball just when you thought you'd figured things out. But here's the good news: understanding intermittent fasting can be a game-changer.

1.1 THE SCIENCE OF INTERMITTENT FASTING: WHAT HAPPENS TO YOUR BODY?

Intermittent fasting (IF) is not about starving yourself, despite what your skeptical friends might think. It's about creating eating windows that allow your body to use its energy more efficiently. The 16/8 method, where you fast for 16 hours and eat during an 8-hour window, is one of the most popular. Then there's the 5:2 method, which involves eating normally for five days and restricting calories for two. And let's not forget the eat-stop-eat method, where you fast for 24 hours once or twice a week. Each method has its own flavor, so to speak, and the flexibility is what makes IF so adaptable.

Fasting isn't just a buzzword; it has deep historical roots. Ancient civilizations practiced fasting for religious and health reasons, long before it became the latest wellness trend. From the Greeks to the Egyptians, fasting was considered a way to purify the body and mind. It's like our ancestors knew something that modern science is only now catching up to. So, when you tell your friends you're trying intermittent fasting, you can also tell them you're partaking in an age-old tradition.

On a cellular level, intermittent fasting does wonders. It triggers a process called autophagy, where your body cleans out damaged cells and regenerates new ones. This is crucial for aging populations because it helps eliminate the cellular junk that accumulates over time. Think of it as a deep-clean for your cells. Then there's insulin sensitivity. Post-menopause, our bodies can become less responsive to insulin, leading to weight gain and increased risk of type 2 diabetes. Intermittent fasting improves insulin sensitivity, helping our cells use glucose more effectively, which means less is stored as fat.

Now, let's talk about inflammation. Chronic inflammation is a silent troublemaker that exacerbates many menopausal symptoms like joint pain and cardiovascular risks. Intermittent fasting helps reduce systemic inflammation, making you feel less like the Tin Man from "The Wizard of Oz" and more like your spry, younger self. And as if that isn't enough, it also helps adapt your metabolic rate. Menopause often slows down metabolism, but intermittent fasting can give it a much-needed boost, aiding in weight management and maintaining steady energy levels.

The psychological benefits are the cherry on top. Many who practice intermittent fasting report improved mental clarity and cognitive function. It's like lifting a fog you didn't even know was there. You might find yourself remembering where you put your keys more often or feeling more focused during tasks. This mental clarity is a game-changer, especially when juggling the various responsibilities that come with this stage of life.

So, there you have it. Intermittent fasting isn't just a new fad; it's a well-researched, historically backed approach to improving your health. It's tailored to meet the unique needs of women over 50, addressing everything from cellular repair to metabolic adaptation. And the best part? It's flexible enough to fit into your life without turning it upside down.

1.2 MENOPAUSE AND METABOLISM: WHAT CHANGES AND WHY

Menopause isn't just about hot flashes and mood swings; it's a hormonal rollercoaster that significantly affects your metabolism. As estrogen and progesterone decline, your metabolism slows down. These hormones, especially estrogen, play a crucial role in regulating metabolic rate. When they plummet, your body becomes less efficient at burning calories. Think of it like a car engine that used to purr like a kitten, but now sputters and coughs. This decline in hormonal levels means your body is more likely to store fat, particularly around the abdomen.

The biological predisposition to accumulate visceral fat during menopause is like a cruel joke played by nature. Visceral fat is the fat that wraps around your internal organs, and it's more dangerous than the subcutaneous fat that sits under your skin. During menopause, the loss of estrogen makes your body more prone to storing fat in this area. Unlike general calorie restriction, which can sometimes lead to muscle loss, intermittent fasting targets visceral fat more effectively. When your body enters a fasting state, it starts to burn stored fat for energy, including that pesky visceral fat.

Thyroid function also takes a hit during menopause. Your thyroid hormones, which are crucial for regulating metabolism, can become imbalanced. This can lead to symptoms like fatigue, weight gain, and depression. Intermittent fasting can help maintain a healthier thyroid hormone balance by reducing inflammation and improving insulin sensitivity. When your body isn't constantly bombarded with food, it has time to reset and heal, which can positively impact thyroid function.

You might be thinking, "Great, so my metabolism is slowing down, and I'm gaining fat. Now what?" The key is adapting your intermittent fasting routine to accommodate these changes. Start with a gentler approach, like the 14/10 method, where you fast for 14 hours and eat during a 10-hour window. Gradually work your way up to longer fasting periods as your body adjusts. Focus on nutrient-dense foods during your eating window to ensure you're getting the vitamins and minerals needed to support your slower metabolism. Foods rich in protein, healthy fats, and fiber can help you feel full longer and stabilize blood sugar levels.

Hormonal changes during menopause don't just affect your metabolism; they also impact your body composition. As estrogen levels drop, you may notice an increase in abdominal fat and a loss of muscle mass. This isn't just about aesthetics; muscle loss can slow your metabolic rate even further. Incorporating strength training into your routine can help maintain muscle mass, which in turn supports a healthier metabolism. Intermittent fasting, combined with resistance exercises, can be a powerful duo in combating these changes.

Menopause also brings changes in appetite and weight management. Hormonal fluctuations can make you feel hungrier and less satisfied after meals. This is where intermittent fasting can be particularly helpful. By restricting your eating window, you're less likely to snack mindlessly throughout the day. You'll find that your body adapts to this new rhythm, and those intense cravings start to diminish. Plus, with fewer opportunities to eat, you naturally consume fewer calories, aiding in weight management.

Understanding these changes is the first step in taking control of your health post-menopause. With the right strategies, intermittent fasting can become a valuable tool in managing weight, boosting energy levels, and improving overall well-being.

1.3 HORMONAL SHIFTS AND THEIR IMPACT ON FASTING

Estrogen is one of those hormones that seems to have a hand in everything, and its fluctuations during menopause can feel like a betrayal. Picture this: your body is suddenly not playing by the rules you've known all your life. These fluctuations can affect how your body responds to fasting. When estrogen levels dip, you might feel hungrier or find it harder to control cravings. But here's the silver lining: intermittent fasting can help regulate these hormonal swings. By establishing a consistent eating window, you can create a rhythm that your body starts to adapt to, helping to stabilize those wild hormonal fluctuations. This can lead to a more balanced feeling overall, reducing those sudden hunger pangs and making it easier to stick to healthy eating habits.

Now, let's talk about cortisol, the stress hormone that seems to spike just when you need it the least. Menopause can send your adrenal glands into overdrive, leading to higher cortisol levels. This can make you feel jittery and stressed, exactly when you're trying to relax. Intermittent fasting can help here too. By giving your body regular breaks from digesting food, you allow your adrenal glands to take a breather. This can help lower cortisol levels, making you feel more at ease. Think of it as a way to hit the reset button on your stress response, giving your body the space it needs to calm down.

Leptin and ghrelin are the dynamic duo of hunger hormones. Leptin tells your brain you're full, while ghrelin signals that you're hungry. During menopause, the balance between these two can get out of whack. You might find yourself feeling hungry even after a meal, or struggling to feel satisfied. Intermittent fasting can help recalibrate this balance. By sticking to specific eating windows, you train your body to release these hormones in a more predictable pattern. Over time, you'll find that your hunger cues become more reliable, making it easier to manage your appetite and avoid overeating.

Customizing your fasting windows to align with your hormonal cycles can make a world of difference. If you find that your energy dips in the afternoon, consider a fasting window that allows you to eat during your high-energy periods and fast during the times when you're less active. This way, you're working with your body's natural rhythms, rather than against them. For example, if you're more energetic in the morning, you might choose an eating window from 8 AM to 4 PM. This allows you to fuel up when you need it most and rest when your body naturally winds down.

Imagine you're attending a family gathering that's scheduled smack in the middle of your fasting window. Instead of stressing out, you can adjust your fasting schedule for that day. Maybe you start your fast a bit earlier or later, allowing you to participate fully without breaking your routine. The key is flexibility. Intermittent fasting isn't a one-size-fits-all approach; it's about finding what works best for you and your unique hormonal landscape.

By understanding how these hormonal shifts impact your body and tailoring your fasting routine accordingly, you can manage the challenges of menopause more effectively. Whether it's balancing hunger hormones, reducing stress, or syncing your eating windows with your energy levels, intermittent fasting offers a versatile toolkit to help you navigate this phase with confidence and ease.

1.4 BENEFITS OF INTERMITTENT FASTING SPECIFICALLY FOR WOMEN OVER 50

As you navigate the wonderful world of intermittent fasting, you'll discover that it's not just about fitting into your favorite pair of jeans again. The benefits go far beyond weight management, especially for women over 50. One of the most exciting areas of research is how intermittent fasting can enhance cognitive function and brain health. Studies have shown that fasting can increase the production of brain-derived neurotrophic factor (BDNF), which supports neuron growth and protection. This is particularly important as we age because lower levels of BDNF are linked to neurodegenerative diseases like Alzheimer's. Imagine feeling sharper and more focused, like you've had a mental tune-up. It's like giving your brain a spa day, every day.

The process of autophagy, which is kicked into high gear during fasting, is a cellular clean-up crew. Your body starts to recycle damaged cells and regenerate healthier ones. This is significant for aging populations because it helps get rid of cellular debris that can lead to chronic illnesses. Think of autophagy as a Marie Kondo for your cells—it keeps what sparks joy (healthy cells) and discards what doesn't (damaged cells). This not only contributes to better health now but also helps in preventing age-related diseases.

Intermittent fasting also holds promise for enhancing longevity and disease prevention. Studies have shown that fasting can activate certain genes that are involved in longevity and stress resistance. For example, research published in journals like "Cell Metabolism" indicates that intermittent fasting can extend lifespan and reduce the onset of age-related diseases in animal models. While we're not mice, the implications are hopeful. It's like having a secret weapon in your wellness arsenal, one that not only helps you live longer, but also live better.

When it comes to mood and emotional well-being, intermittent fasting can be a game-changer. Many women report feeling a sense of emotional stability and reduced anxiety. This is partly because fasting helps regulate cortisol levels, the stress hormone we mentioned earlier. By giving your body a break from constant digestion, you allow your adrenal glands to relax, which can lead to a calmer mind. It's like finding an oasis of peace in the middle of a chaotic day.

Improved cardiovascular health is another significant benefit. Fasting has been shown to lower blood pressure and improve cholesterol levels, which are crucial for menopausal women who are at a higher risk of heart diseases. By reducing bad cholesterol (LDL) and increasing good cholesterol (HDL), intermittent fasting helps keep your arteries clear and your heart healthy. It's like giving your cardiovascular system a much-needed tune-up.

Bone density maintenance is yet another area where intermittent fasting can make a difference. As we age, maintaining bone density becomes increasingly important to prevent osteoporosis. While more research is needed, some studies suggest that intermittent fasting can help in maintaining bone health by reducing inflammation and improving nutrient absorption. Think of it as giving your bones the support they need to stay strong and resilient.

Quality of life improvements round out the benefits of intermittent fasting. Many women report better sleep patterns, which in turn, enhance overall vitality. When you sleep better, you wake up feeling refreshed, ready to tackle the day with newfound energy. Enhanced mood, steady energy levels, and a general sense of well-being are all part of the package. It's like upgrading your life to a premium version, where every day feels a bit brighter and more manageable.

1.5 ADDRESSING COMMON MENOPAUSAL SYMPTOMS WITH INTERMITTENT FASTING

Hot flashes and night sweats can feel like your body's way of playing a cruel joke. One minute you're perfectly fine, and the next you're fanning yourself like you're in the Sahara. The stabilization of insulin levels through intermittent fasting can be a game-changer here. High insulin levels can exacerbate these symptoms, making you feel hotter and sweatier. By fasting, you're giving your body a break from constant insulin production, which can help stabilize it. Additionally, fasting reduces systemic inflammation, another culprit behind these annoying symptoms. Imagine fewer nights waking up drenched and more nights of uninterrupted sleep. It's not magic, but it's pretty close.

Weight management during menopause can feel like trying to climb a mountain in flip-flops. The usual tricks just don't work the way they used to. Intermittent fasting can help here by providing a structured eating pattern that naturally reduces calorie intake without the need for obsessive counting. The 16/8 method, for example, limits your eating window, making it easier to avoid late-night snacking. Over time, this leads to a natural reduction in calorie intake, helping you manage your weight more effectively. The key is consistency; sticking to a fasting routine can help you see gradual, sustainable weight loss.

16/8 Fasting
Fasting Window: **16 hours**
Eating Window: **8 hours**

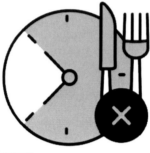

How it works:
- Skip Breakfast: Start your day with water or black coffee/tea.
- Early Lunch: Have your first meal around noon.
- Early Dinner: Finish your last meal by 8 PM

Potential Benefits:
- Weight Loss
- Improved Insulin Sensitivity
- Reduced Inflammation
- Cellular Repair

Energy levels can be a rollercoaster during menopause. One moment you're ready to conquer the world, and the next you're searching for the nearest couch. Intermittent fasting can help stabilize your energy levels throughout the day. This is partly due to improved mitochondrial function. Mitochondria are the power-houses of your cells, and fasting helps them work more efficiently. When your cells can produce energy more effectively, you feel more energetic and less prone to those mid-afternoon slumps. It's like giving your body a more efficient engine, one that keeps you going strong all day long.

Mood swings during menopause can make you feel like you're living with an unpredictable roommate. One minute you're laugh-ing, the next you're in tears. The hormonal balance achieved through intermittent fasting can help stabilize your mood. By regulating insulin and cortisol levels, fasting helps to keep your hormones in check. This means fewer mood swings and a more stable emotional state. Imagine feeling more balanced and in control, able to handle whatever life throws your way with a calm and steady demeanor.

There's a myth that older women shouldn't fast because it can lead to muscle loss. Let's debunk that right now. Intermittent fasting, when done correctly, does not cause muscle wasting. In fact, fasting can help preserve muscle mass by promoting the release of human growth hormone (HGH). Pairing fasting with strength training exercises can further ensure that you maintain, or even build, muscle mass. So, you can put aside those fears and embrace fasting as a safe and effective tool for maintaining muscle health.

Safety and efficacy are often concerns, especially when trying something new. Rest assured, intermittent fasting is safe for older adults. Numerous scientific studies support its benefits and safety profile. The key is to listen to your body and start slowly. Begin with shorter fasting windows and gradually extend them as your body adapts. Consulting with a healthcare provider can also provide personalized guidance, ensuring that fasting is appropriate for your individual health needs.

Nutrient intake is another concern. How do you ensure you're getting all the nutrients you need? The answer lies in well-planned meal choices. Focus on nutrient-dense foods during your eating windows. Think fresh fruits, vegetables, lean proteins, and healthy fats. These choices provide the vitamins and minerals your body needs to thrive. By making mindful food choices, you can support your health while reaping the benefits of intermittent fasting.

Fasting and bone health is another area of concern, especially with the risk of osteoporosis. The good news is that intermittent fasting does not negatively affect bone density. In fact, some studies suggest that fasting can help reduce inflammation, which is beneficial for bone health. Ensuring adequate calcium and vitamin D intake during your eating windows can further support bone density. So, you can fast confidently, knowing your bones are in good hands.

1.6 THE SCIENCE OF FASTING: BENEFITS BEYOND WEIGHT LOSS

Menopause shakes up your metabolism like a snow globe. One minute, everything's settled, and the next, it's all up in the air. Aging slows metabolic rates, which means your body becomes less efficient at burning calories. This isn't just about weight; it's about energy balance. Remember when you could eat a whole birthday cake and not feel like you needed a nap afterward? Those days may be behind us, but intermittent fasting can help restore some of that metabolic flexibility. By alternating between periods of eating and fasting, your body learns to switch between using glucose and stored fats for energy more efficiently. This metabolic flexibility can make it easier to manage your weight and keep your energy levels steady throughout the day.

Intermittent fasting also impacts where and how your body stores fat. During menopause, many women notice an increase in visceral fat—the kind that wraps around your internal organs and is more harmful than the fat under your skin. Unlike general calorie restriction, which can sometimes lead to muscle loss, inter-mittent fasting targets visceral fat more effectively. This means you're not just shedding pounds; you're losing the kind of fat that poses the greatest health risks. Think of it as a targeted fat reduction strategy that works from the inside out.

Several studies have explored the impact of intermittent fasting on post-menopausal women's metabolism. For instance, a study published in "Obesity" found that women who practiced intermit-tent fasting experienced significant reductions in visceral fat and improvements in insulin sensitivity. Another study in "Cell Metabolism" showed that intermittent fasting could help regulate hormones that control hunger and satiety, making it easier to maintain a healthy weight. These findings are not just numbers on a page; they're real-world evidence that intermittent fasting can make a significant difference in your health.

Beyond the physical benefits, intermittent fasting can also enhance cognitive function. Research has shown that intermittent fasting increases the production of brain-derived neurotrophic factor (BDNF), which supports neuron growth and protection. This is crucial for aging populations because lower levels of BDNF are linked to neurodegenerative diseases like Alzheimer's. Imagine feeling sharper, more focused, and mentally agile, as if you've had a mental tune-up. It's like giving your brain a fresh start, every day.

Cardiovascular health is another area where intermittent fasting shines. Studies have shown that fasting can lower blood pressure and improve cholesterol levels, both of which are crucial for menopausal women at higher risk of heart diseases. By reducing bad cholesterol (LDL) and increasing good cholesterol (HDL), intermittent fasting helps keep your arteries clear and your heart healthy. It's like giving your cardiovascular system a much-needed tune-up, ensuring that it runs smoothly for years to come.

Bone density is a significant concern for women over 50, as the risk of osteoporosis increases with age. While more research is needed, some studies suggest that intermittent fasting can help maintain bone health by reducing inflammation and improving nutrient absorption. Ensuring adequate calcium and vitamin D intake during your eating windows can further support bone density. This means you can fast confidently, knowing your bones are in good hands.

The holistic improvements in quality of life that come with intermittent fasting are the icing on the cake. Many women report better sleep patterns, enhanced mood, and increased overall vitality. When you sleep better, you wake up feeling refreshed, ready to tackle the day with newfound energy. Enhanced mood, steady energy levels, and a general sense of well-being are all part of the package. It's like upgrading your life to a premium version, where every day feels a bit brighter and more manageable.

By understanding these benefits, it's clear that intermittent fasting offers far more than just weight loss. It's a multifaceted approach to health that can significantly improve your quality of life, especially during and after menopause. Whether it's boosting your metabolism, enhancing cognitive function, or improving cardiovascular health, intermittent fasting provides a holistic path to feeling better, living healthier, and aging gracefully.

2

PREPARING FOR YOUR FASTING JOURNEY

I magine standing on the edge of a diving board. You're about to take the plunge into something new and exciting, but also a bit daunting. That's how starting intermittent fasting might feel. But don't worry, you're not alone. Think of this chapter as your swim coach, guiding you through the basics to ensure you're ready to make a splash.

2.1 ESSENTIAL MEDICAL CHECKS BEFORE STARTING

First things first: before you dive in, it's crucial to consult with a healthcare provider. You wouldn't start a road trip without checking your car, right? The same goes for your body. A healthcare provider can assess any pre-existing conditions that might affect your ability to safely practice intermittent fasting. For instance, conditions like diabetes, thyroid disorders, or even a history of eating disorders require special attention. Your healthcare provider can help tailor a plan that's safe and effective for you.

Baseline health metrics are the next step. These are the health stats that provide a snapshot of where you're starting from. Think of them as the "before" photo in your health journey. Important metrics to monitor include blood glucose levels, cholesterol levels, and blood pressure. Knowing these numbers not only helps you track your progress but also ensures you're fasting safely. Blood glucose levels, for instance, can tell you how well your body is managing sugar. High levels might indicate insulin resistance, a common issue post-menopause, which intermittent fasting can help improve. Cholesterol levels and blood pressure are also vital, especially since menopause can increase your risk of cardiovascular diseases.

Medication adjustments are another critical area to discuss with your healthcare provider. If you're managing chronic conditions like hypertension or diabetes, the timing and dosage of your medications might need tweaking. For example, some medications need to be taken with food, which can be tricky when you're fasting. Your healthcare provider can guide you on how to adjust your medication schedule to fit your fasting routine. This might mean taking your meds during your eating window or making other adjustments to ensure you're not compromising your health.

Checklist: Pre-Fasting Medical Check-Up

- **Consult Your Healthcare Provider:** Discuss your plan to start intermittent fasting and get personalized advice.
- **Baseline Health Metrics:** Record your blood glucose levels, cholesterol levels, and blood pressure.
- **Review Medications:** Discuss potential adjustments to medication timing and dosage.

Armed with this information, you can tailor your fasting regimen to your specific health needs and limitations. This personalized approach ensures that you're not just following a generic plan, but one that's designed with you in mind. It's like having a custom-made dress—it fits perfectly and makes you feel fabulous.

So, before you start skipping meals or changing your eating patterns, take the time to get these medical checks done. It's a small step that makes a big difference in ensuring your intermittent fasting journey is not only effective but also safe. Now, with your health baseline established, and any necessary medication adjustments made, you're ready to dive into the world of intermittent fasting with confidence and clarity.

2.2 MENTAL PREPARATION FOR A FASTING LIFESTYLE

Starting intermittent fasting is a bit like preparing for a marathon. It's not just about the physical aspects; the mental game is equally important. Picture this: you've decided to try intermittent fasting, but the idea of skipping meals feels daunting. That's perfectly normal. Mental readiness for this lifestyle change requires a shift in how you think about food and fasting. Begin by setting your intention. Why are you doing this? Is it to feel more energetic, manage your weight, or perhaps reduce menopausal symptoms? Clearly defining your "why" can provide motivation when the going gets tough.

Now, let's talk about the elephant in the room—hunger and cravings. These are not just physical sensations but psychological challenges. You might find yourself staring longingly into the pantry, thinking about that chocolate bar hidden behind the cereal. One effective strategy is to distract yourself. Engage in activities that keep your mind off food. Take a walk, read a book, or call a friend. Another trick is to drink water or herbal tea.

Sometimes what we perceive as hunger is actually thirst. If cravings hit hard, try deep breathing exercises. Inhale deeply, hold, and exhale slowly. This can help calm your mind and reduce the urge to eat.

Building mental resilience is like strengthening a muscle. It takes practice and patience. Start by setting small, achievable goals. Maybe begin with a 12-hour fast and gradually extend it. Celebrate your successes, no matter how small. Did you make it through your first 14-hour fast? Fantastic! Give yourself credit. Also, anticipate setbacks. There will be days when you feel tempted to break your fast early. Instead of seeing it as a failure, view it as a learning experience. What triggered the urge to eat? Was it stress, boredom, or social pressure? Understanding these triggers can help you develop strategies to manage them in the future.

Emotional fluctuations are part and parcel of dietary changes, especially during fasting. You might feel irritable one moment and euphoric the next. This is where mindfulness comes in handy. Practice being present in the moment often. If you feel a wave of irritation, acknowledge it without judgment. Say to yourself, "I'm feeling irritable right now, and that's okay." This simple act of acknowledgment can lessen the emotional charge. Journaling is another powerful tool. Write down your thoughts and feelings about fasting. What challenges are you facing? How do you feel physically and emotionally? This can provide valuable insights and help you manage your emotional landscape better.

To make this process even more engaging, let's do a quick exercise.

Reflective Exercise: Understanding Your Triggers

Take a few minutes to jot down answers to these questions:

1. What are my main motivations for trying intermittent fasting?
2. What activities can I do to distract myself from cravings?
3. What triggers my cravings or the urge to eat outside of my eating window?
4. How can I celebrate my small wins to stay motivated?
5. How do I typically handle emotional fluctuations, and what new strategies can I try?

Reflecting on these questions can give you a clearer picture of your mental landscape and prepare you for the psychological aspects of fasting. Remember, mental preparation is just as crucial as the physical adjustments. With the right mindset, you can navigate the ups and downs of intermittent fasting more smoothly and effectively.

2.3 SETTING REALISTIC GOALS AND EXPECTATIONS

Setting realistic goals for intermittent fasting can feel like a balancing act. You want to aim high, but you also need to keep your feet on the ground. That's where SMART goals come in handy. These are Specific, Measurable, Achievable, Relevant, and Time-bound targets that align with your health objectives and lifestyle. For instance, instead of saying, "I want to lose weight," you could set a goal like, "I aim to lose 10 pounds over the next three months by following a 16/8 fasting schedule." This goal is specific (lose 10 pounds), measurable (you can track your weight), achievable (10 pounds in three months is realistic), relevant (it aligns with your health goals), and time-bound (three months).

Setting SMART goals can make the daunting task of intermittent fasting seem more manageable and less overwhelming.

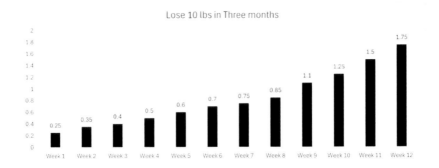

Adjusting your expectations is another crucial part of the process. When you start intermittent fasting, you might feel like a super-hero for the first few days, but then reality hits. Hunger pangs, mood swings, and low energy can make you question your decision. It's important to understand that these initial challenges are normal. Your body is adjusting to a new routine, and it needs time to adapt. Benefits like weight loss, improved energy levels, and better mood might not be noticeable immediately. Typically, you might start seeing changes within a few weeks, but significant results can take a couple of months. Patience is the key point. Don't expect overnight miracles. Instead, focus on the gradual, sustainable progress you're making.

Personalizing your fasting goals is essential because no two bodies are the same. Your health status, lifestyle, and menopausal symptoms will influence how you approach intermittent fasting. For example, if you have a busy work schedule, a 16/8 fasting window might be more practical than the 5:2 method. If you're dealing with severe menopausal symptoms like hot flashes or night sweats, you might need to adjust your fasting schedule to ensure you're getting enough nutrients to manage these symptoms. The goal is to find a fasting plan that fits seamlessly into your life, rather than trying to fit your life around a rigid fasting schedule.

Monitoring your progress is more than just stepping on the scale. While weight is an important metric, it's not the only one you should consider. Pay attention to how you feel overall. Are your energy levels improving? Do you feel more mentally clear? Are your menopausal symptoms becoming more manageable? Keeping a journal can be a helpful way to track these changes. Note down your energy levels, mood, sleep quality, and any changes in your symptoms. This can provide a more holistic view of your progress and keep you motivated even when the scale isn't moving as fast as you'd like.

Creating a checklist can also be beneficial. Include items like "Track my weight weekly," "Note changes in energy levels," and "Record mood and symptom changes." This helps you stay organized and focused on your goals. It's also a tangible way to see your progress over time, which can be incredibly motivating. Remember, the goal of intermittent fasting isn't just to lose weight; it's to improve your overall health and well-being. Keeping track of all these different metrics can give you a clearer picture of how far you've come and where you need to adjust.

As you set your goals and adjust your expectations, keep in mind that intermittent fasting is a flexible tool. It's not a one-size-fits-all solution, and it's okay to tweak your approach as you go along. The key is to stay committed and be patient with yourself. With time, you'll find a rhythm that works for you, and the benefits will start to unfold.

2.4 CREATING A SUPPORTIVE ENVIRONMENT FOR FASTING

You know how it goes: you've decided to start intermittent fasting, and suddenly, everyone around you becomes a food critic. Your spouse wonders why you're skipping breakfast, your friends think you're on some bizarre diet, and your kids are convinced you're starving yourself. Educating family and friends about intermittent fasting is crucial to garner support and reduce potential friction during meal times. Start by explaining the why behind your decision. Share the benefits you hope to achieve, like improved energy, better mood, and manageable weight. Use simple language and relatable examples. Maybe even show them a few articles or studies—nothing too heavy, just enough to back up your choice. This way, they're more likely to support you and less likely to offer you pancakes at 7 AM.

Joining fasting communities can also provide a wealth of support and motivation. These can be online forums, social media groups, or even local meet-ups. In these communities, you'll find people who are going through the same challenges and triumphs as you. They can offer tips, share recipes, and provide that extra bit of encouragement when you're feeling tempted to raid the fridge. Plus, hearing other people's success stories can be incredibly motivating. It's like having a group of cheerleaders who understand exactly what you're going through. And let's face it, sometimes we all need a little extra cheerleading.

Setting up your physical environment to support your fasting goals is another key step. Start in the kitchen. Remove or hide the foods that are your biggest temptations. Out of sight, out of mind, right? Stock up on healthy foods that you can enjoy during your eating window. Think fresh fruits, vegetables, lean proteins, and whole grains. Organize your pantry so that healthy options are easy to grab. You might even create a special section in your fridge or pantry for your fasting-friendly foods. This way, when it's time to eat, you're not rummaging through bags of chips and cookies to find something healthy.

Incorporating fasting into your daily routine is all about finding a rhythm that works for you. If you have a busy schedule, plan your fasting and eating windows around your most active times. For instance, if you're not a morning person, you might choose to skip breakfast and have your eating window start around noon. This way, you can enjoy dinner with your family without feeling deprived. On the flip side, if you're an early riser, you might prefer an earlier eating window that allows you to have breakfast and lunch, then fast through dinner. The key is to make intermittent fasting fit seamlessly into your life, rather than trying to force your life to fit around a rigid fasting schedule.

Also, consider your social activities. If you know you have a dinner date or a social event coming up, plan your fasting schedule accordingly. Maybe you adjust your eating window for that day so you can enjoy the event without breaking your fast. Flexibility is your friend here. You don't have to be perfect; you just have to be consistent.

Creating a supportive environment for fasting involves educating those around you, finding your tribe, setting up your space for success, and integrating fasting into your daily life in a way that feels natural and sustainable. It's about making small, thoughtful changes that support your goals and help you stay on track.

2.5 THE ROLE OF HYDRATION AND SUPPLEMENTS

Imagine your body as a well-oiled machine. Just like any machine, it needs the right fluids to keep running smoothly. During intermittent fasting, hydration becomes even more crucial. When you're fasting, your body isn't getting the usual hydration from food, so you need to drink more water to compensate. Hydration affects everything from your metabolism to your detoxification processes. Think of water as the fuel that keeps your engine running. Without it, you might feel sluggish, tired, or even dizzy. Aim to drink at least eight glasses of water a day, and more if you're active or the weather is hot. Herbal teas and infused water can be great additions if plain water feels too monotonous.

Now, let's talk about electrolytes. These are minerals like sodium, potassium, magnesium, and calcium that help maintain the balance of fluids in your body. When you're fasting, your body continues to use and lose these essential electrolytes through sweat and urine. An imbalance can lead to dehydration, muscle cramps, and even heart palpitations. So, how do you keep your electrolytes in check? One way is through your diet during your eating window. Foods like bananas, avocados, nuts, and leafy greens are rich in electrolytes. Another option is to use electrolyte supplements, especially if you're doing longer fasts. Look for supplements without added sugars to keep it clean and healthy.

Speaking of supplements, let's dive into which ones might be beneficial during intermittent fasting. Magnesium is a big one. It helps with muscle function, reduces cramps, and can even improve sleep quality. Omega-3 fatty acids are another excellent choice. They support heart health, reduce inflammation, and can help with mood regulation. Multivitamins can be a good catch-all to ensure you're getting all the essential nutrients, especially if your diet isn't always perfect. If you're worried about bone health, a calcium supplement might be beneficial too. Always consult with your healthcare provider before starting any new supplements to make sure they're right for you.

Timing your supplements is also crucial for maximizing their effectiveness. Some supplements are best taken with food to improve absorption. For instance, fat-soluble vitamins like A, D, E, and K should be taken during your eating window with a meal that contains some healthy fats. On the other hand, some supplements like magnesium can be taken before bed to help with sleep. If you're taking a multivitamin, the morning might be the best time, as it can boost your energy levels throughout the day. Electrolyte supplements can be taken during your eating window to ensure you're replenishing any lost minerals.

Maintaining hydration and a balanced intake of electrolytes and supplements can make your intermittent fasting experience much smoother and more enjoyable. By paying attention to these details, you're setting yourself up for success, ensuring that your body gets the support it needs to thrive.

2.6 THE FUTURE OF INTERMITTENT FASTING: EMERGING RESEARCH

If you think intermittent fasting is just a passing trend, think again. The future is bright and filled with exciting possibilities. Emerging research is diving into how intermittent fasting impacts genetic expression and longevity genes. For instance, studies are showing that fasting can activate certain genes associated with longevity and disease resistance. Imagine having a genetic switch that, when flipped, could help you live longer and healthier. It's like finding the fountain of youth but in your own DNA. Researchers are looking into how fasting influences the expression of genes related to aging, cellular repair, and stress resistance. This could mean that fasting isn't just about weight loss, but about turning back the biological clock.

Personalized fasting protocols are another fascinating development. We all know that one-size-fits-all rarely works, especially when it comes to health. Scientists are now exploring how personalized fasting plans can be created based on your genetic makeup, lifestyle, and specific health needs. Think of it as a tailor-made suit but for your diet. This approach could revolutionize health optimization by making fasting more effective and accessible for everyone. For example, if your genes indicate a higher risk for diabetes, a personalized fasting plan could be designed to help regulate blood sugar more efficiently. This customization ensures that you're not just following a generic plan, but one that's specifically designed for your unique body and health goals.

Technological advancements are also playing a huge role in the future of intermittent fasting. Gone are the days of manually tracking your fasting and eating windows with a pen and paper. Today, there are numerous apps designed to help you monitor your fasting schedule, track your progress, and even remind you when it's time to start or stop eating. Wearable devices like smartwatches are taking it a step further by providing real-time data on your physiological changes during fasting. These gadgets can monitor your heart rate, sleep patterns, and even stress levels, giving you a comprehensive view of how fasting is impacting your body. It's like having a personal health coach on your wrist, guiding you every step of the way.

The global health implications of widespread intermittent fasting adoption are also worth noting. Imagine a world where obesity and metabolic syndrome are no longer epidemics. Intermittent fasting has the potential to combat these conditions on a large scale. Research shows that fasting can help reduce body weight, improve glucose metabolism, and lower the risk of cardiovascular diseases. These benefits don't just apply to individuals; they can have a profound impact on public health. By reducing the incidence of obesity and related conditions, we could see a significant decrease in healthcare costs and an overall improvement in quality of life for many people. It's like a domino effect: one healthy habit leading to widespread benefits.

As we look to the future, it's clear that intermittent fasting is more than just a diet trend. It's a powerful tool that can transform health on multiple levels. From genetic research to personalized plans and technological advancements, the possibilities are endless. This chapter has given you a glimpse into what's on the horizon, but the real excitement lies in how these advancements will shape your own health journey.

With these insights in mind, we'll move forward to explore the practical aspects of implementing intermittent fasting in your daily life. Up next, we'll delve into the various fasting methods and how to choose the one that fits you best.

3

FASTING METHODS AND PERSONALIZATION

Picture this: you're sitting at your kitchen table, sipping a cup of herbal tea, and flipping through yet another health magazine. You come across an article on intermittent fasting and think, "Could this really work for me?" You've tried countless diets and exercise routines, only to find that post-menopausal body of yours just isn't responding like it used to. The good news? Intermittent fasting offers a variety of methods that can be personalized to fit your lifestyle and health needs.

3.1 EXPLORING DIFFERENT FASTING WINDOWS AND THEIR EFFICACY

There are several popular fasting windows, and each has its own structure and benefits. Let's start with the 16/8 method. This approach involves fasting for 16 hours and eating during an 8-hour window. For many, this means skipping breakfast and having your first meal around noon, then eating until 8 PM. The 16/8 method is popular because it's relatively easy to adjust your daily routine to fit this schedule. It allows you to enjoy social meals, like lunch and dinner, without feeling like you're missing out.

Next up is the 5:2 method. This involves eating normally for five days of the week and drastically reducing calorie intake (to about 500-600 calories) for the remaining two days. The 5:2 method can be particularly effective for weight management because it combines periods of normal eating with calorie restriction. It's like having your cake and eating it too—just not every day. This method is appealing because it allows for flexibility. You can choose which two days to restrict calories based on your schedule, making it easier to adhere to.

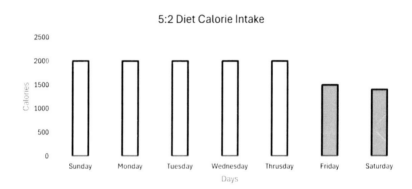

Then there's the eat-stop-eat method, which involves fasting for a full 24 hours once or twice a week. For example, if you finish dinner at 7 PM, you wouldn't eat again until 7 PM the next day. This method might sound intense, but it can be incredibly effective for weight loss and metabolic health. The 24-hour fast gives your body a break from constant digestion, allowing it to focus on cellular repair and fat burning. Plus, knowing you only have to fast once or twice a week can make the rest of the week feel like a breeze.

The effectiveness of each fasting window varies, particularly for women over 50. The 16/8 method is often praised for its simplicity and sustainability. Studies have shown that this method can help improve insulin sensitivity, which is crucial for managing weight and preventing type 2 diabetes. The 5:2 method, on the other hand, has been found to be effective for reducing visceral fat, the kind that wraps around your internal organs and poses significant health risks. Given that post-menopausal women are more prone to accumulating visceral fat, the 5:2 method can be particularly beneficial.

The eat-stop-eat method is backed by research showing significant benefits for metabolic health. A study published in "Cell Metabolism" found that 24-hour fasting can improve glucose metabolism and reduce inflammation. This is particularly relevant for women over 50, who often face increased inflammation and metabolic challenges. By giving your body a full day to reset, you can enhance your overall health and well-being.

Real-life examples bring these methods to life. Take Susan, a 54-year-old teacher who struggled with weight gain and low energy post-menopause. She started with the 16/8 method, skipping breakfast and eating from noon to 8 PM. Within a few weeks, she noticed a significant boost in her energy levels and a gradual decrease in her weight. Then there's Janet, a 60-year-old retiree who tried the 5:2 method. She found that the flexibility of choosing her two fasting days made it easy to stick to her routine. Over three months, Janet lost 15 pounds and reported feeling more vibrant and less bloated.

Research supports these personal testimonies. The National Institutes of Health has documented the benefits of intermittent fasting for metabolic health, particularly in older adults. Studies have shown improvements in insulin sensitivity, reductions in inflammation, and better weight management outcomes. These findings are not just numbers on a page; they translate into real-world benefits that can make a significant difference in your life.

Incorporating intermittent fasting into your routine doesn't have to be complicated. By understanding the different fasting windows and their benefits, you can choose a method that fits your lifestyle and health needs. Whether it's the simplicity of the 16/8 method, the flexibility of the 5:2 method, or the metabolic boost of the eat-stop-eat method, there's a fasting window that's right for you. So, grab that cup of herbal tea and consider which method might be your perfect fit.

3.3 TAILORING YOUR FASTING PLAN TO YOUR LIFE

When it comes to tailoring your fasting plan, the first step is assessing your lifestyle needs. Think about your typical day. Are you an early bird or a night owl? Do you have a bustling work schedule, or are your days more relaxed? Maybe you have social obligations, like weekly family dinners or book club meetings, that you wouldn't dream of missing. All these factors play a role in choosing the right fasting method. For example, if your mornings are hectic, you might find it easier to skip breakfast and start your eating window later. Conversely, if you enjoy a leisurely breakfast but find evenings are more flexible, an earlier eating window could work better for you.

Flexibility in fasting is crucial, especially during periods of high-stress or social events. Life happens, and it doesn't always align perfectly with our plans. The beauty of intermittent fasting is its adaptability. If you have a special event coming up, like a wedding or a holiday, you can adjust your fasting schedule without guilt. Maybe you extend your eating window for that day or shift your fasting hours to accommodate a late dinner. The key is to be kind to yourself and understand that flexibility is part of the process. Stressful periods at work or home may also require a temporary adjustment. If fasting feels like an added stressor during these times, consider shortening your fasting window or taking a brief break. Your mental health matters just as much as your physical health.

Incorporating your personal preferences and eating habits is another essential factor. If you love a hearty breakfast but can easily skip dinner, then tailor your fasting plan to suit this preference. The goal is to make the fasting experience enjoyable and sustainable. Consider your food preferences, too. If you're a fan of big family meals, plan your eating window to include these times. This way, you're not sitting at the dinner table with a glass of water while everyone else enjoys a feast. Adjusting your fasting windows to accommodate your lifestyle makes it easier to stick with the plan long-term. For instance, if you have a 9-to-5 job, an eating window from 12 PM to 8 PM might be perfect, allowing you to have lunch at work and dinner at home without feeling rushed.

Adjusting as you go is a natural part of intermittent fasting. Your life isn't static, and your fasting plan shouldn't be either. Periodically reassess your fasting regimen to ensure it still aligns with your lifestyle and health goals. Maybe you started with the 16/8 method and found it works well, but your new job requires you to start early and finish late. In that case, you might switch to a 14/10 schedule that better fits your new routine. Similarly, if you notice changes in your health status, like a new medical diagnosis or a shift in medication, it's essential to adjust your fasting plan accordingly. Your body's needs can change over time, and being flexible with your fasting approach ensures you continue to reap the benefits without compromising your well-being.

For instance, let's say you've been following a particular fasting schedule for a few months, but you're not seeing the results you hoped for. It's time to reassess. Maybe try a different fasting window or method. If you've been doing the 16/8, perhaps the 5:2 method might kickstart your progress. The key is to listen to your body and be willing to make changes as needed. Remember, intermittent fasting is not a one-size-fits-all approach. What works for one person might not work for another, and that's perfectly okay. The goal is to find a plan that fits seamlessly into your life and supports your health goals.

Periodic reassessment also allows you to stay in tune with your body's signals. If you start feeling unusually fatigued, irritable, or notice other negative symptoms, it might be a sign that your current fasting plan needs tweaking. Don't be afraid to experiment and find what works best for you. Your fasting plan should evolve with you, adapting to the ebb and flow of your life. So, as you continue on this path, stay flexible, be patient with yourself, and remember that adjustments are a natural part of the process.

3.4 COMBINING FASTING WITH YOUR CURRENT DIET

You've found your fasting window, and now you're wondering how to combine it with your current diet without feeling like you're depriving yourself. The great news is that intermittent fasting is incredibly versatile and can be adapted to fit various dietary preferences and requirements. Whether you're plant-based, follow a Mediterranean diet, or lean towards a low-carb lifestyle, there's a way to make intermittent fasting work for you.

If you're plant-based, focus on incorporating a variety of whole foods during your eating window. Think legumes, whole grains, vegetables, fruits, nuts, and seeds. These foods are not only nutrient-dense, but also provide the fiber necessary for good digestion.

Plant-based proteins like tofu, tempeh, and lentils can help keep you full and support muscle health. On the other hand, if you follow a Mediterranean diet, you're already on the right track. This diet emphasizes healthy fats, lean proteins, and plenty of fruits and vegetables. During your eating window, focus on meals rich in olive oil, fish, nuts, and whole grains. These foods align well with the health benefits of intermittent fasting, such as improved heart health and reduced inflammation.

For those who prefer a low-carb approach, intermittent fasting can enhance the benefits of a ketogenic or Atkins-style diet. Aim to consume high-quality fats like avocado, coconut oil, and nuts, along with proteins such as chicken, beef, and fish. Low-carb vegetables like spinach, kale, and broccoli can round out your meals, providing essential vitamins and minerals. The combination of low-carb eating and intermittent fasting can help your body enter ketosis more efficiently, promoting fat burning and boosting energy levels.

Timing your nutrient intake is crucial for maximizing the health benefits of intermittent fasting. Prioritize protein intake during your eating window to support muscle health, especially as muscle mass tends to decrease with age. Consuming protein-rich foods like eggs, lean meats, dairy, or plant-based proteins in each meal can help maintain muscle mass and aid in recovery. Carbohydrates should be timed around your most active parts of the day to ensure you have the energy you need. For example, if you exercise in the morning, breaking your fast with a balanced meal containing carbs can replenish your glycogen stores and aid in muscle recovery.

Intermittent fasting can also impact digestion and nutrient absorption. When you're not constantly feeding your body, your digestive system gets a much-needed break. This can improve the efficiency of nutrient absorption when you do eat. However, it's important to choose easy-to-digest foods to avoid overwhelming your stomach. Start your eating window with lighter meals and gradually move to more substantial ones. For instance, breaking your fast with a smoothie or a light salad can ease your digestive system back into action, followed by a more substantial meal like grilled chicken with quinoa and vegetables.

Here are some example meal plans to get you started, tailored for post-menopausal women. For a plant-based diet, you might start your eating window with a spinach and berry smoothie, followed by a lunch of lentil soup with a side of quinoa salad. Dinner could be a hearty vegetable stir-fry with tofu and a handful of nuts for a snack. If you prefer the Mediterranean diet, break your fast with Greek yogurt topped with berries and honey, enjoy a lunch of grilled salmon with a side of tabbouleh, and finish with a dinner of roasted chicken, sautéed greens, and a drizzle of olive oil. For a low-carb approach, start with a breakfast of scrambled eggs with avocado, have a lunch of grilled steak with a side of cauliflower rice, and end your day with a dinner of baked cod and a generous helping of leafy greens.

Incorporating intermittent fasting into your diet doesn't mean you have to overhaul your entire eating plan. It's about making thoughtful choices that align with your personal preferences and nutritional needs. By focusing on nutrient timing, optimizing digestion, and selecting foods that support your overall health, you can make intermittent fasting a seamless and beneficial part of your life.

3.5 ADJUSTMENTS FOR ENERGY MAINTENANCE DURING FASTING

Managing energy levels during fasting can feel like trying to balance on a tightrope. One minute, you're walking tall, and the next, you're wobbling. But don't worry; there are strategies to help maintain your energy throughout the fasting period. Staying hydrated is the first and most crucial step. Water is your best friend here. It keeps your metabolism humming and helps prevent the dreaded energy dip. Consider adding a slice of lemon or a few cucumber slices to your water for a refreshing twist. Herbal teas are another great option. They're caffeine-free, so you can sip on them throughout the day without worrying about disrupting your sleep later.

Adjusting the timing of your fasting window can also make a significant difference. If you find yourself dragging in the afternoon, consider shifting your eating window to earlier in the day. For example, if you're currently doing a 16/8 fast from noon to 8 PM, try moving it to 10 AM to 6 PM. This way, you're fueling your body earlier, which can help sustain your energy levels throughout the day. Strategic caffeine use can also be beneficial. A cup of black coffee or green tea during your fasting hours can provide a gentle energy boost without breaking your fast. Just remember to keep it moderate to avoid any jittery side effects.

Choosing nutrient-dense foods during your eating window is crucial for maintaining energy levels. Focus on balanced meals that include a mix of protein, healthy fats, and complex carbohydrates. For instance, a meal of grilled chicken, quinoa, and steamed vegetables provides a good balance of macronutrients. Protein is particularly important for muscle health, while healthy fats like avocado and nuts can help keep you satiated. Complex carbs, such as sweet potatoes or whole grains, provide sustained energy without causing a spike in blood sugar. Avoid empty calories and sugary snacks, as they can lead to energy crashes and leave you feeling worse.

Supplements can also play a role in sustaining energy during fasting. B vitamins are known for their energy-boosting properties. They help convert food into energy and support brain function. You might consider a B-complex supplement, which includes all the essential B vitamins. Amino acids, the building blocks of protein, can also be beneficial. They help maintain muscle mass and support recovery, especially if you're engaging in physical activity. Another supplement to consider is magnesium, which can help with muscle function and reduce fatigue. Always consult with your healthcare provider before starting any new supplements to ensure they're right for you.

Aligning more demanding physical and cognitive activities with your eating window can make a big difference. If you know you have a busy afternoon ahead, try scheduling your eating window to end just before these activities. This way, you're fueled and ready to take on the tasks at hand. For instance, if you have a workout planned, aim to complete it shortly after your first meal. This ensures you have the energy to perform well and recover effectively. Similarly, if you have a mentally demanding project, scheduling it after a meal can help you stay focused and productive. This alignment can help you make the most out of your fasting and eating periods.

Recognizing signals that indicate a need for adjustments in your fasting approach is essential for maintaining optimal energy levels. If you start feeling unusually fatigued, dizzy, or irritable, it might be a sign that your current fasting plan needs tweaking. Pay attention to these cues and be willing to make changes as needed. For example, if you're experiencing afternoon energy crashes, consider shifting your eating window earlier or incorporating more nutrient-dense foods into your meals. Another sign to watch for is difficulty sleeping. If fasting is disrupting your sleep, it might be worth adjusting your fasting hours or ensuring you're getting enough nutrients during your eating window.

Maintaining energy levels during fasting is a balancing act, but with the right strategies, it's entirely manageable. Stay hydrated, choose nutrient-dense foods, consider supplements, and align your activities with your eating window. And most importantly, listen to your body's signals. It's okay to make adjustments as you go along. This flexibility ensures that you can sustain your fasting practice while feeling energized and vibrant.

3.6 WHEN TO MODIFY YOUR FASTING PLAN

Listening to your body is like having a heart-to-heart with an old friend. It knows what you need, even when you're too busy to notice. As you practice intermittent fasting, it's crucial to pay attention to the physical and mental feedback your body gives you. Feeling unusually fatigued or irritable? These might be signs that your current fasting plan needs a tweak. Maybe the fasting period is too long, or perhaps you need to adjust the frequency. The key is to make changes that maintain the health benefits of fasting while minimizing any risks. Shorten your fasting window if you feel constantly drained, or try reducing the number of fasting days if they seem overwhelming. Remember, your body is your best guide; listen to it.

Health changes can also necessitate modifications to your fasting plan. Life happens, and as we age, new medical diagnoses or changes in medication can pop up unexpectedly. Maybe you're diagnosed with a condition that requires you to take medication with food, or perhaps your doctor prescribes a new medication that affects your appetite. These changes require a reassessment of your fasting schedule. For instance, if you're now required to take medication in the morning with food, you might need to

our eating window to accommodate this. Always consult
our healthcare provider when making these changes to
e that your fasting plan remains safe and effective.

Sometimes, despite your best efforts, the current fasting plan just isn't delivering the results you hoped for. Maybe the scale isn't budging, or you're experiencing negative symptoms like headaches or digestive issues. It's important to identify these signs and understand that they might indicate the need for adjustments. For example, if you're not seeing weight loss, consider whether your eating window needs to be shorter or if the foods you're consuming during your eating window are nutrient-dense and balanced. If you're experiencing digestive issues, you might need to ease into fasting more gradually or adjust the types of foods you're eating. The goal is to find a balance that supports your health and well-being without causing adverse effects.

Your health goals and life circumstances are not static; they evolve over time. Maybe you initially started intermittent fasting to lose weight, but now you're more focused on improving your energy levels or managing a specific health condition. As your goals change, your fasting plan should adapt accordingly. If you've reached your weight loss goal and now want to focus on muscle maintenance, you might adjust your fasting schedule to ensure you're getting enough protein throughout the day. Similarly, if a new job or family obligation changes your daily routine, your fasting plan should be flexible enough to accommodate these changes. The idea is to keep your fasting plan aligned with your current needs and objectives, ensuring it continues to support your health in the best way possible.

Take, for example, Joan. She started intermittent fasting with the 16/8 method to lose weight and had great success initially. However, after a few months, she hit a plateau and started feeling more tired than usual. Listening to her body, Joan realized she needed to make some changes. She shortened her fasting window to 14/10 and included more nutrient-dense foods in her meals. She also started taking a B-complex supplement to boost her energy levels. These adjustments helped her break through the plateau and regain her energy. Joan's experience highlights the importance of being flexible and willing to adapt your fasting plan as needed.

So, as you continue with intermittent fasting, remember that flexibility is your friend. Listen to your body, consult with your healthcare provider, and be willing to make adjustments based on your health status, goals, and life circumstances. Intermittent fasting is not a one-size-fits-all approach; it's a dynamic process that evolves with you. By staying attuned to your body's signals and making thoughtful adjustments, you can ensure that your fasting plan remains effective and supportive of your overall health and well-being.

With this in mind, you're now ready to explore how intermittent fasting integrates with physical activity, ensuring you get the most out of both worlds.

4

NUTRITIONAL STRATEGIES FOR SUSTAINABLE FASTING

You've just finished a delightful lunch and are feeling pretty good about your fasting routine. But then the questions start to creep in. What should you be eating during your eating window to maximize the benefits of intermittent fasting? How do you ensure you're getting all the nutrients you need, especially as a woman over 50? Let's dig into the nitty-gritty of macronutrients and micronutrients to help you craft a diet that supports your health, energy, and overall well-being.

4.1 MACRONUTRIENTS AND MICRONUTRIENTS: WHAT YOU NEED TO KNOW

Balancing macronutrients is like conducting an orchestra. You need the right mix of proteins, fats, and carbohydrates to create a harmonious symphony that supports your health. Proteins are the strings, providing the backbone of muscle maintenance and repair. As we age, muscle mass naturally declines, which can lead to weight gain and decreased strength. Ensuring an adequate protein intake is crucial. Aim for about 1.0 to 1.2 grams of protein per kilogram of body weight per day. This translates to incorporating lean meats, dairy products, legumes, and nuts into your meals. Proteins not only help preserve muscle mass but also contribute to satiety, keeping you feeling full longer and preventing unnecessary snacking.

Carbohydrates are the woodwinds, providing the primary energy source your body needs to keep moving. But not all carbs are created equal. Focus on quality carbohydrates like whole grains, vegetables, fruits, and legumes. These foods are rich in essential nutrients and dietary fiber, which aid in digestive health and regulate blood sugar levels. Fiber is particularly important because it helps you feel full and satisfied, reducing the urge to overeat. Aim for carbohydrates to make up about 45% to 65% of your total energy intake. This balance ensures you're getting enough energy to fuel your daily activities without causing spikes and crashes in blood sugar.

Fats are the brass section, essential for absorbing fat-soluble vitamins and supporting cell function. As the risk of heart disease increases during post-menopause, it's important to focus on healthy fats. These include monounsaturated and polyunsaturated fats found in olive oil, avocados, nuts, seeds, and fatty fish. These fats help reduce inflammation and support heart health. Aim for fats to make up about 20% to 35% of your total daily calories, while minimizing saturated and trans fats. Including healthy fats in your diet not only supports your heart but also helps you feel satisfied and energized.

Now, let's talk about the percussion section—micronutrients. These are the vitamins and minerals that, though needed in smaller amounts, are crucial for your overall health. For women over 50, certain micronutrients become even more important. Calcium and vitamin D are essential for maintaining bone health and preventing osteoporosis. As estrogen levels decline, the risk of bone density loss increases, making these nutrients vital. Magnesium is another key player, supporting muscle function, reducing cramps, and improving sleep quality. Vitamin B12 is crucial for energy levels and cognitive function, as absorption can decrease with age. Incorporating foods rich in these micronutrients, such as dairy products, leafy greens, nuts, seeds, and fortified cereals, can help maintain your health.

Timing your nutrient intake can enhance their absorption and utilization. For instance, consuming protein-rich foods shortly after breaking your fast can support muscle repair and growth. Carbohydrates are best consumed earlier in the day to provide sustained energy. Healthy fats can be included throughout your eating window to aid in satiety and nutrient absorption. Consider pairing calcium-rich foods with vitamin D sources to improve absorption. For example, have a glass of fortified orange juice with your breakfast or a serving of salmon with your dinner. This strategic timing ensures that your body gets the most out of the nutrients you consume.

Finally, diet diversity is essential for covering all your nutritional bases. Think of your diet as a colorful palette, with each food bringing its own unique benefits. Incorporating a variety of foods ensures you get a comprehensive nutrient profile, reducing the need for excessive reliance on supplements. Rotate your protein sources between lean meats, plant-based options, and dairy. Mix up your carbohydrate choices with different whole grains, fruits, and vegetables. Include a range of healthy fats from various nuts, seeds, and oils. This variety not only keeps your meals interesting but also supports overall health by providing a wide range of nutrients.

To help you get started, here's a quick checklist:

Nutrient Timing Checklist:

- **Protein:** Consume shortly after breaking your fast to support muscle repair.
- **Carbohydrates:** Focus on earlier in the day for sustained energy.
- **Healthy Fats:** Include throughout your eating window for satiety and nutrient absorption.
- **Calcium and Vitamin D:** Pair together for optimal absorption, such as dairy with fortified foods.

Balancing your macronutrients and ensuring you get essential micronutrients can make a significant difference in how you feel and function. By paying attention to what you eat and when you eat it, you're setting yourself up for a successful and sustainable fasting routine.

4.2 PLANNING YOUR MEALS: WHAT TO EAT DURING YOUR EATING WINDOW

When structuring meals for optimal nutrition, think of your plate as a well-rounded team, each member playing a crucial role. Start by ensuring a balanced intake of macronutrients—proteins, fats, and carbohydrates. Proteins should be a focal point, helping to maintain muscle mass and keep you feeling full longer. Lean meats, fish, beans, and legumes are excellent choices. Carbohydrates should come from whole grains, vegetables, and fruits, providing steady energy without causing spikes in blood sugar. Healthy fats, such as those found in avocados, nuts, and olive oil, support cellular functions and help you absorb essential vitamins. Portion control is key; use smaller plates or bowls to help regulate portion sizes and prevent overeating. Distribute your meals evenly throughout your eating window to maintain steady energy levels and hormonal balance. For example, if your eating window is from 12 PM to 8 PM, consider having a meal at noon, a snack around 3 PM, and dinner at 7 PM.

Incorporating whole foods into your meals is like giving your body the VIP treatment. Whole foods are minimally processed and closer to their natural state, which means they retain more nutrients. Fresh fruits, vegetables, whole grains, lean proteins, and healthy fats should form the backbone of your diet. Processed foods, on the other hand, often contain high levels of sugars, unhealthy fats, and artificial additives that can disrupt your metabolic health. Instead of grabbing a bag of chips, opt for a handful of nuts or a piece of fruit. Whole foods not only provide essential nutrients but also help keep you full and satisfied, reducing the likelihood of cravings and overeating. Think of meals like a colorful salad with mixed greens, cherry tomatoes, cucumbers, grilled chicken, and a drizzle of olive oil. Pair it with a side of quinoa and a piece of fruit for a well-rounded, nutrient-dense meal that fuels your body.

Hydration plays a vital role in digestion and metabolism, and it's essential to integrate fluids into your meal times effectively. Drinking water before and during meals can aid digestion and help you feel full, preventing overeating. However, be mindful not to drink excessive amounts right before or during meals, as it can dilute digestive enzymes and hinder the digestive process. Aim to sip water throughout the day and include hydrating foods like cucumbers, watermelon, and leafy greens in your diet. Herbal teas and infused water can also add variety and make hydration more enjoyable. Remember, staying hydrated supports your body's functions and can help maintain energy levels, especially during your fasting periods. Aiming for about eight glasses of water a day is a good starting point, but listen to your body and adjust as needed based on your activity level and climate.

Creating a meal schedule that distributes nutrient intake optimally throughout your eating window can make fasting more manageable and effective. Start your eating window with a balanced meal that includes proteins, healthy fats, and complex carbohydrates to break your fast gently and provide sustained energy. For example, a bowl of Greek yogurt topped with berries, nuts, and a drizzle of honey can be a great option. Follow this with a nutrient-dense lunch, such as a quinoa salad with mixed vegetables, chickpeas, and a light vinaigrette. In the afternoon, a small snack like apple slices with almond butter can help bridge the gap until dinner. Your final meal of the day should be satisfying but not overly heavy, like a piece of grilled salmon with a side of roasted sweet potatoes and steamed broccoli. This structure helps maintain steady energy levels and supports overall health.

Consider the transition into and out of the fasting state. Pre-fasting meals should be balanced and not overly heavy, setting you up for a comfortable fasting period. Foods rich in fiber and protein can help keep you full longer. For example, a meal of chicken breast with a side of brown rice and steamed vegetables can be filling without being too heavy. Post-fasting meals should ease you back into eating gently, avoiding foods that are too rich or heavy. Start with something light, like a smoothie with spinach, banana, and a scoop of protein powder, before moving on to a more substantial meal. This approach helps your body transition smoothly and supports digestive health.

By paying attention to meal structure, incorporating whole foods, staying hydrated, and planning your meal schedule thoughtfully, you can make the most of your eating window and support your intermittent fasting goals.

4.3 ANTI-INFLAMMATORY FOODS THAT ENHANCE FASTING BENEFITS

Imagine you're setting a beautiful table with foods that not only taste great but also work wonders for your health. Anti-inflammatory foods are the unsung heroes of your diet, especially when paired with intermittent fasting. Think of turmeric, berries, nuts, and leafy greens as your go-to ingredients. Turmeric contains curcumin, a powerful anti-inflammatory compound. Berries like blueberries and strawberries are rich in antioxidants that help combat inflammation. Nuts, such as almonds and walnuts, provide healthy fats and antioxidants. Leafy greens like spinach and kale are packed with vitamins that support overall health. These foods can naturally complement the anti-inflammatory effects of intermittent fasting, making your meals both delicious and beneficial.

At the cellular level, these anti-inflammatory foods work in fascinating ways. Curcumin in turmeric, for instance, inhibits molecules that play a significant role in inflammation, like nuclear factor kappa B (NF-kB). This can help reduce the risk of chronic diseases such as arthritis and heart disease. The antioxidants in berries neutralize free radicals, unstable molecules that can damage cells and lead to inflammation. Nuts contain omega-3 fatty acids, which are known to reduce the production of inflammatory molecules. Leafy greens are rich in vitamins A and C, both of which have anti-inflammatory properties. By reducing inflammation, these foods improve joint health, cardiovascular function, and overall well-being. It's like giving your body a daily dose of TLC.

Integrating these anti-inflammatory foods into your daily meals doesn't have to be a chore. Start your day with a smoothie that includes spinach, berries, and a dash of turmeric. For lunch, a salad with mixed greens, walnuts, and a light vinaigrette can be both satisfying and nutritious. Snack on a handful of almonds or a piece of fruit. Dinner could feature a piece of grilled salmon (another excellent source of omega-3s), accompanied by a side of sautéed kale. Experimenting with spices like turmeric in soups and stews can add both flavor and health benefits. The key is to make these foods a regular part of your diet, ensuring they're both appetizing and nutritionally beneficial. Over time, you'll find that these small changes can make a big difference in how you feel.

Common inflammation-related issues, such as arthritis and metabolic syndrome, are often part of the post-menopausal landscape. Arthritis can make your joints feel like rusty hinges, and metabolic syndrome can leave you feeling sluggish and prone to weight gain. Anti-inflammatory foods can play a crucial role in addressing these concerns. Omega-3 fatty acids, found in fatty fish and nuts, can help reduce joint pain and stiffness. Berries and leafy greens can improve blood sugar regulation, helping to manage metabolic syndrome. Including these foods in your diet can enhance the quality of life and make fasting more effective. Think of it as adding a little extra armor to your health arsenal.

For those dealing with arthritis, incorporating turmeric into your diet can provide relief. A study published in the "Journal of Medicinal Food" found that curcumin had significant anti-inflammatory and antioxidant properties, making it effective in managing arthritis symptoms. Similarly, a diet rich in omega-3 fatty acids can help reduce joint inflammation and pain. If metabolic syndrome is a concern, focusing on fiber-rich foods like fruits, vegetables, and whole grains can help regulate blood sugar levels and improve insulin sensitivity. A balanced diet that includes anti-inflammatory foods can make a significant impact on your overall health, making intermittent fasting not just a diet but a holistic approach to wellness.

By focusing on anti-inflammatory foods and understanding their mechanisms of action, you can make informed choices that enhance the benefits of intermittent fasting. Integrating these foods into your daily meals can help manage common post-menopausal health concerns, improving your quality of life and making fasting a more effective and enjoyable experience. So, let's sprinkle some turmeric, toss in some berries, and embrace the power of anti-inflammatory foods in our daily diet.

4.4 RECIPES FOR THE EATING WINDOW: SIMPLE AND NUTRITIOUS

Creating recipes that are both nutritious and simple to prepare is key, especially when you're juggling a busy lifestyle and a limited eating window. Start by focusing on ingredients that are easy to find and don't require hours in the kitchen. Think of recipes like a symphony, where each ingredient plays its part in creating a harmonious and satisfying meal. For breakfast, how about a quick avocado toast? Mash a ripe avocado, spread it on whole-grain toast, sprinkle some chia seeds, and add a dash of lemon juice. It's loaded with healthy fats, fiber, and a burst of vitamins, making it a perfect way to break your fast.

For lunch, a Mediterranean quinoa salad can be a winner. Cook some quinoa and let it cool. Mix in chopped cucumbers, cherry tomatoes, red onions, Kalamata olives, and feta cheese. Drizzle with olive oil and a splash of red wine vinegar. This salad is packed with protein, healthy fats, and complex carbs that will keep you satisfied. Dinner could be a simple sheet pan meal. Arrange chicken breasts, sweet potatoes, and broccoli on a baking sheet, drizzle with olive oil, sprinkle with your favorite herbs, and bake until everything is cooked through. This one-pan meal is easy to prepare and clean up, making it ideal for busy evenings.

Adapting these recipes to cater to different tastes, dietary restrictions, and seasonal availability is easier than you might think. If you're vegetarian, swap the chicken in the sheet pan meal for tofu or tempeh. Lactose intolerant? Skip the feta in the quinoa salad and add some extra olives or roasted chickpeas for that salty kick. Seasonal ingredients can also keep your meals fresh and exciting. In the summer, you might add fresh strawberries to your quinoa salad, while in the winter, roasted butternut squash could be a delightful addition. Being flexible with your ingredients ensures that your meals remain enjoyable and sustainable, no matter the season or dietary preference.

Meal prepping can be a game-changer, especially when you're trying to stick to a nutritious fasting regimen. Spend a couple of hours on the weekend prepping your meals for the week. Cook a batch of quinoa, grill some chicken, and chop a variety of vegetables. Store everything in airtight containers in the fridge. This way, when it's time to eat, you can quickly assemble a healthy meal without the temptation to reach for convenience foods. For breakfast, pre-portion ingredients for smoothies into freezer bags. In the morning, just add a bag to your blender with some almond milk, and you're good to go. For lunch, prepare mason jar salads. Layer your ingredients, with the dressing at the bottom and greens at the top, to keep everything fresh until you're ready to eat.

Having a few go-to recipes that you can prepare in advance will save you time and stress. A big pot of vegetable soup can be portioned out for lunches or dinners. It's easy to make, full of nutrients, and can be customized with whatever vegetables you have on hand. Another great option is a frittata. Whisk eggs with a splash of milk, pour over sautéed vegetables in a skillet, and bake until set. Cut into wedges and store in the fridge for a quick breakfast or lunch. These meals are not only nutritious, but also convenient, making it easier to stick to your fasting plan.

By focusing on simple, nutritious recipes and incorporating meal prepping into your routine, you can ensure that you always have healthy options available. This reduces the likelihood of reaching for less nutritious convenience foods and helps you stay on track with your fasting goals. So, get creative in the kitchen, experiment with different ingredients, and enjoy the process of nourishing your body with delicious, healthy meals.

4.5 UNDERSTANDING AND MANAGING CRAVINGS

Cravings can feel like an insistent toddler tugging at your sleeve —persistent and hard to ignore. But where do these cravings come from? They're not just about hunger. Physiologically, cravings often stem from your brain's reward system. When you eat something tasty, your brain releases dopamine, the "feel-good" hormone. This can create a cycle where you crave more of that food to get the same dopamine hit. Psychologically, cravings can be linked to emotions like stress, boredom, or even happiness. Differentiating between hunger and cravings is crucial. Hunger is your body's way of signaling it needs fuel, while cravings are more about wanting something specific, often for emotional or sensory satisfaction. Intermittent fasting can affect these sensations, sometimes intensifying cravings initially as your body adjusts, but over time, helping to regulate them as your body finds a new rhythm.

Managing cravings doesn't have to feel like a Herculean task. One practical strategy is distraction. When a craving hits, engage in an activity that absorbs your attention. Go for a walk, call a friend, or dive into a hobby. These distractions can help reduce the intensity of the craving. Ensuring adequate nutrient intake during your eating window can also play a significant role. When your body gets the vitamins and minerals it needs, cravings often diminish. Mindful eating practices can make a big difference too. Slow down, savor each bite, and pay attention to your body's signals of fullness and satisfaction. This mindfulness can help you feel more in control and less likely to give in to cravings. Another tip is to stay hydrated. Sometimes what we perceive as a craving is actually thirst. Drinking a glass of water can help mitigate this.

When it comes to handling cravings, having healthy alternatives on hand can be a lifesaver. If you're craving something sweet, reach for a piece of fruit instead of a candy bar. Berries or apple slices with a bit of nut butter can satisfy your sweet tooth while keeping you on track with your nutritional goals. Crave something crunchy? Try a handful of nuts or some air-popped popcorn instead of chips. If you're in the mood for something creamy, Greek yogurt with a drizzle of honey and a sprinkle of nuts can hit the spot. These alternatives allow you to indulge without derailing your dietary goals, making it easier to stick with intermittent fasting.

Over time, as your body adapts to intermittent fasting, you may notice a reduction in the frequency and intensity of cravings. This is partly because your body becomes more efficient at using stored energy and balancing hunger hormones like ghrelin and leptin. Ghrelin signals hunger, while leptin signals fullness. As your body gets used to fasting, these hormones start to regulate better, leading to fewer cravings. Long-term management of cravings involves fostering healthy eating habits. Incorporating a variety of nutrient-dense foods into your diet can help keep cravings at bay. Regular meal planning and prepping can ensure you always have healthy options available, reducing the temptation to reach for less nutritious foods. Consistency is key; the more you practice these habits, the easier they become, creating a sustainable lifestyle that supports your health and well-being.

Understanding the sources of cravings and implementing strategies to manage them can make your intermittent fasting experience smoother and more enjoyable. By distinguishing between hunger and cravings, using practical tips to handle them, and choosing healthy alternatives, you can maintain control over your dietary choices. Over time, your body will adapt, and you'll find that cravings become less of a challenge, allowing you to focus on the broader benefits of intermittent fasting.

As we wrap up this chapter, remember that managing cravings is a journey of self-awareness and practice. Embrace the process, make adjustments as needed, and celebrate your progress. Next, we'll explore the integration of physical activity to complement your fasting routine, enhancing your overall health and vitality.

5

INTEGRATING PHYSICAL ACTIVITY

You know those days when you finally muster the energy to put on your workout gear, only to find yourself standing in the middle of the living room wondering, "Now what?" Well, you're not alone. Many of us have been there, especially when trying to juggle the complexities of post-menopausal life with a new intermittent fasting routine. But fear not! This chapter is here to guide you through the maze of integrating physical activity with intermittent fasting, ensuring you get the most out of both worlds.

5.1 THE BEST TYPES OF EXERCISE DURING INTERMITTENT FASTING

Aligning your exercise routines with your fasting and eating windows can make all the difference in the world. Imagine starting your day with a brisk walk or a gentle yoga session before your first meal. This way, you're utilizing your body's stored energy (mostly from fat), which can enhance fat burning without overly depleting your glycogen stores. Think of it as giving your metabolism a little nudge to get going in the morning. Timing is everything here. Doing moderate aerobic activities, like walking, cycling, or a light jog, during the fasting period can help you tap into fat stores more effectively. These exercises are gentle enough to keep you from feeling drained, but effective enough to promote fat burning.

During your eating window, it's prime time for more intense activities. This is when your body has the fuel it needs to power through a workout and recover efficiently. Strength training, for instance, is highly beneficial when done after you've had a meal. Lifting weights or doing resistance exercises during this period can help maximize muscle synthesis and repair. It's like fueling up your car before a long drive—you'll get much farther and perform better when your tank is full. The key is to find a balance that works for you, ensuring you're not overexerting yourself during fasting but still getting the most out of your workouts during your eating window.

Safety considerations are paramount, especially if you're new to fasting or have pre-existing health conditions. Start slow and listen to your body. If you're not used to exercising on an empty stomach, begin with shorter, low-intensity sessions and gradually build up. Hydration is crucial. Drink plenty of water before, during, and after your workouts to prevent dehydration, which can be more pronounced when fasting. Also, be mindful of signs of overexertion, such as dizziness, excessive fatigue, or muscle cramps. These can be indicators that you need to dial back the intensity or adjust your fasting schedule.

Activity Journal: Tracking Your Progress

Keeping a journal of your physical activities can be incredibly helpful. Note down the type of exercise, duration, and how you felt before, during, and after the workout. This can help you identify the best times to exercise and make necessary adjustments to your routine.

- **Date:**
- **Type of Exercise:**
- **Duration:**
- **Energy Levels (Before/During/After):**
- **Notes:**

Types of beneficial exercises during fasting include activities like walking, cycling, and low-impact aerobics. These exercises promote fat burning without depleting your glycogen stores too quickly. Walking is particularly great because it's easy on the joints and can be done almost anywhere. Cycling provides a bit more intensity while still being manageable. Low-impact aerobics can be a fun way to get your heart rate up without the jarring effects of high-impact exercises. The goal is to keep moving without pushing your body to the point of exhaustion.

Exercise timing is another critical factor. To maximize fat loss, aim to do your aerobic activities during the fasting period, when your body is more likely to burn stored fat for energy. For example, a morning walk before breakfast can set a positive tone for the day and help you burn fat more efficiently. On the other hand, to maximize recovery and muscle synthesis, schedule your strength training sessions during your eating window. This way, your body has the nutrients it needs to repair and build muscle. A late-afternoon or early evening workout can be ideal, followed by a protein-rich meal to support recovery.

Safety considerations cannot be overstated. Ensure you're not overexerting yourself, especially if you're new to fasting or have any health conditions. Start with low-intensity exercises and gradually increase the intensity as your body adapts. Always stay hydrated, as dehydration can occur more easily when fasting. If you experience any signs of overexertion or dehydration, such as dizziness, extreme fatigue, or muscle cramps, stop exercising and consult with a healthcare provider if necessary. These precautions will help you integrate physical activity into your intermittent fasting routine safely and effectively.

5.2 LOW-IMPACT EXERCISES FOR SUSTAINABLE HEALTH

Low-impact exercises are the unsung heroes of the fitness world, especially for women over 50. These exercises, such as swimming, cycling, and walking, offer a plethora of benefits without putting undue stress on your joints. Imagine gliding through a pool, feeling weightless and free, while giving your muscles a thorough workout. Swimming is fantastic for cardiovascular health and muscle toning, all while being gentle on your knees and hips. Cycling, whether on a stationary bike or a scenic trail, provides an excellent aerobic workout that builds leg strength and boosts cardiovascular endurance. Walking, the simplest of them all, can be done anywhere and requires no special equipment. It's perfect for maintaining daily activity levels and can be easily incorporated into your routine.

Incorporating low-impact exercises into your daily life doesn't have to be a chore. Think of it as weaving small yet meaningful activities into the fabric of your day. For instance, take the stairs instead of the elevator, park farther from the store entrance, or enjoy a leisurely walk after dinner. These small changes can add up over time, making a significant difference in your overall fitness. Set a daily step goal and use a pedometer or a smartphone app to track your progress. You might be surprised at how quickly those steps add up! If you enjoy socializing, consider joining a local walking group or a community swim class.

Exercising with others can make the activity more enjoyable and keep you motivated.

Effective low-impact workout routines can vary depending on your fitness level and personal preferences. For beginners, a simple routine might include a 10-minute warm-up of gentle stretching followed by 20 minutes of brisk walking. If you're feeling up to it, you can add a few intervals of faster walking to get your heart rate up. For those with access to a pool, swimming laps for 30 minutes is a great full-body workout. You can alternate between different strokes, like freestyle, backstroke, and breast-stroke, to keep things interesting. If you prefer cycling, a 30-minute ride at a moderate pace is excellent for building endurance. You can also try a low-impact aerobics class, either in-person or online, which combines gentle movements with music for a fun and energizing workout. These routines are easy to customize based on your fitness level and can be adjusted as you progress.

Adjusting the intensity and duration of low-impact exercises is crucial for continued progress. Start with what feels comfortable and gradually increase the intensity as your fitness improves. For instance, if you're walking, try adding a few hills or increasing your pace. If you're cycling, adjust the resistance on your stationary bike or explore more challenging outdoor routes. The key is to listen to your body and make changes in small incre-ments. If you're new to swimming, start with shorter sessions and gradually add more laps as your stamina builds. It's important to challenge yourself, but not to the point of discomfort or injury. Over time, you'll notice improvements in your endurance, strength, and overall fitness, which can be incredibly motivating.

Low-impact exercises are a fantastic way to stay active and healthy without putting unnecessary stress on your joints. They're suitable for daily routines and can be easily integrated into your life. By choosing activities you enjoy, setting realistic goals, and gradually increasing the intensity, you can maintain a consistent and enjoyable exercise routine. Whether it's a morning swim, an afternoon bike ride, or an evening walk, these activities can help you stay fit, healthy, and energized. So, lace up those walking shoes, hop on that bike, or dive into the pool, and enjoy the benefits of low-impact exercise for sustainable health.

5.3 BALANCING CARDIO AND STRENGTH TRAINING

Maintaining muscle mass during and after menopause is like keeping your car's engine in top shape. You wouldn't ignore a check engine light, so why overlook your muscle health? As we age, muscle mass naturally declines, which can lead to a slower metabolism and increased risk of osteoporosis. Strength training is your ally here. It not only helps maintain muscle mass but also boosts metabolic health and supports bone density. Think of it as giving your bones and muscles the reinforcement they need to stay strong and resilient. By incorporating regular strength training, you're setting yourself up for better weight management and overall health.

Designing a balanced exercise routine that includes both cardio and strength training can feel like putting together a puzzle. The pieces need to fit together just right to create a complete picture of health. Start by assessing your current fitness level and health goals. If you're aiming for overall fitness, a good rule of thumb is to dedicate about 150 minutes per week to moderate aerobic activity and include strength training exercises at least two days a week. This balance ensures you're getting the cardiovascular benefits of cardio while also building and maintaining muscle through strength training. Tailor the intensity and duration based on your energy levels and personal preferences. For example, if you find high-intensity workouts too taxing, opt for moderate-intensity exercises that are easier to sustain.

A sample weekly exercise plan might look something like this: On Monday, start with a brisk 30-minute walk followed by 20 minutes of light strength training exercises like body weight squats, lunges, and push-ups. Tuesday could be a rest day or a gentle yoga session to keep things flexible. On Wednesday, return to a more intense cardio session, like a 45-minute bike ride or a swim, paired with some core exercises. Thursday could be another strength training day, focusing on different muscle groups with exercises like dumbbell rows, shoulder presses, and leg presses. Friday might be perfect for a low-impact cardio session, such as a 30-minute elliptical workout or a dance class. The weekend can be a mix of activities you enjoy—perhaps a long hike on Saturday and a rest or light stretching on Sunday. This plan ensures a balanced approach, keeping your body engaged without overwhelming it.

Listening to your body's responses to different exercises is crucial. Your body has its own way of communicating, and it's important to pay attention. If you notice persistent soreness, fatigue, or lack of motivation, it might be a sign that you need to adjust the balance between cardio and strength training. For instance, if you're feeling worn out after a few weeks, try reducing the frequency of high-intensity cardio sessions and adding more rest or low-impact activities. On the flip side, if you're not seeing the strength gains you hoped for, consider incorporating more resistance exercises or increasing the weight you're lifting. The key is to find a routine that challenges you but also allows for recovery and adaptation.

Another important aspect is to adapt your routine based on your fasting schedule. If you find that your energy levels are lower during fasting periods, schedule more intense workouts during your eating windows. This ensures you have the fuel needed for optimal performance and recovery. For example, plan your strength training sessions after a meal to take advantage of the nutrients available for muscle repair and growth. Cardio sessions can be scheduled earlier in the day if you prefer to fast in the evening, ensuring you still get the metabolic benefits without overexerting yourself.

Balancing cardio and strength training can be a rewarding and effective way to maintain your health. By focusing on muscle maintenance, designing a balanced routine, and listening to your body's signals, you can create a fitness plan that supports your overall well-being. Whether it's lifting weights, walking, cycling, or dancing, the combination of these activities will help you stay fit, strong, and energized.

5.4 YOGA AND FLEXIBILITY WORKOUTS FOR WOMEN OVER 50

Picture yourself on a yoga mat, sunlight streaming through the window, and the gentle hum of nature in the background. Yoga and flexibility training offer a treasure trove of benefits, especially for women over 50. Improved range of motion is one of the biggest perks. As we age, our joints can become stiff, making everyday activities more challenging. Yoga helps keep those joints limber, allowing you to move with more ease and less discomfort. And let's not forget the mental benefits. Yoga is a wonderful stress reducer. The combination of deep breathing and mindful move-ment can help lower cortisol levels, leaving you feeling more relaxed and centered. Enhanced mental clarity is another gift from yoga. By focusing on your breath and movements, you create a meditative state that clears the mental clutter, making you more present and focused in your daily life.

When it comes to tailoring yoga practices for fasting periods, it's all about energy conservation and gentle stimulation. During fasting, your energy reserves might be lower, so opt for types of yoga that are less intense, like Hatha or Yin yoga. These styles focus on slow, deliberate movements and long-held poses that promote relaxation and flexibility without draining your energy. On the flip side, during your eating windows, you can incorporate more dynamic styles like Vinyasa or Ashtanga, which help stimulate digestion and circulation. These more vigorous practices can help your body process the nutrients you consume more efficiently. Think of it as giving your digestive system a little nudge to get things moving.

Let's talk about yoga routines for different times of the day. In the morning, a gentle routine can help wake up your body and mind. Start with some deep breathing exercises, followed by gentle stretches like Cat-Cow, Downward Dog, and Child's Pose. These poses help loosen up your spine and get your blood flowing. An afternoon routine can be a bit more dynamic, incorporating poses like Warrior I and II, Tree Pose, and Bridge Pose. These poses build strength and balance while giving you a mid-day energy boost. In the evening, opt for restorative poses like Legs-Up-The-Wall, Reclining Bound Angle Pose, and Corpse Pose. These calming poses help you unwind and prepare for a restful night's sleep.

Integrating mindfulness and meditation into your yoga practice can amplify the benefits of both intermittent fasting and physical exercise. Mindfulness is all about being present in the moment, fully aware of your thoughts, feelings, and bodily sensations. By incorporating mindfulness into your yoga practice, you create a deeper connection between your mind and body. Start your practice with a few minutes of seated meditation, focusing on your breath. As you move through your poses, maintain this awareness, paying attention to how your body feels in each position. End your practice with a few more minutes of meditation, allowing yourself to fully relax and absorb the benefits of your practice.

Meditation, in particular, can be a powerful tool for managing the mental and emotional aspects of fasting. When those hunger pangs hit, instead of reaching for a snack, take a few moments to meditate. Focus on your breath, allowing the sensation of hunger to pass without judgment. This can help you develop a more mindful relationship with food and reduce the urge to eat out of boredom or stress. Over time, you'll find that meditation becomes a natural part of your fasting routine, helping you stay calm, focused, and in control.

Imagine starting your day with a few Sun Salutations, moving with the rhythm of your breath, feeling your body wake up and come alive. In the afternoon, you might take a break from your busy day to practice a few standing poses, grounding yourself and finding balance amidst the chaos. As evening falls, you roll out your mat for a restorative practice, allowing your body and mind to unwind, releasing the stresses of the day. This seamless integration of yoga and mindfulness into your daily routine can transform your fasting experience, making it not just a dietary change but a holistic approach to better health and well-being.

5.5 MONITORING YOUR PHYSICAL RESPONSE TO EXERCISE WHILE FASTING

Keeping tabs on how your body responds to exercise while fasting is a bit like being your own health detective. You need to pay attention to several key indicators to ensure you're not pushing yourself too hard. First and foremost, keep an eye on your heart rate. If you're exercising and your heart rate skyrockets or stays elevated longer than usual, it might be a sign to dial back the intensity. A good rule of thumb is to stay within your target heart rate zone, which is typically 50-85% of your maximum heart rate. Calculating this is simple: subtract your age from 220, and then multiply that number by 0.50 and 0.85 to find your range.

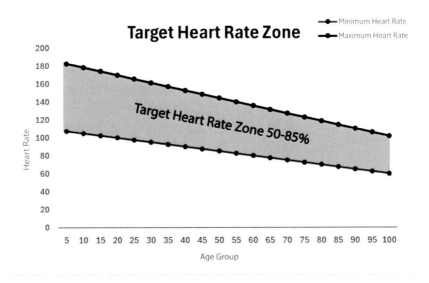

Hydration status is another crucial indicator. During fasting, your body isn't getting fluids from food, so you need to be extra vigilant about drinking water. Dehydration can sneak up on you, leading to dizziness, fatigue, and even muscle cramps. Check the color of your urine; a pale yellow indicates proper hydration, while darker shades mean you need to drink more water. Energy levels are also telling. If you find yourself dragging through workouts or feeling unusually tired afterward, it's a cue that you might need to adjust your fasting or exercise routine. Consistency is key, but so is listening to what your body tells you.

Modern technology can be a fantastic ally in monitoring these indicators. Fitness trackers and heart rate monitors are excellent tools to keep tabs on your vitals. Devices like Fitbits, Apple Watches, or Garmin watches can track your heart rate, steps, and even your sleep patterns. These gadgets often come with apps that let you log your water intake and set hydration reminders. They can also track your energy expenditure, giving you a clearer picture of how your body is responding to both fasting and exercise. If you're more into old-school methods, a simple notebook can work wonders. Jot down your daily exercise routines, how you felt before and after, and any physical symptoms you noticed.

Interpreting body signals is where the detective work gets interesting. Fatigue, for instance, isn't just about feeling tired; it's your body's way of saying it needs more recovery time. If you're constantly feeling worn out, it might be a sign that your exercise intensity is too high or that you're not getting enough nutrients during your eating window. Dizziness is another red flag. If you feel lightheaded during a workout, it's a strong indicator that you need to stop, hydrate, and possibly eat something. Excessive sweating can also be a clue. While sweating is normal during exercise, an unusual amount could mean you're overexerting yourself or that your body is struggling to cool down. These signals are your body's way of communicating its needs, so it's crucial to pay attention and respond accordingly.

Making feedback-driven adjustments to your exercise routine is the final piece of the puzzle. Based on the data you collect and the signals your body sends, you can tweak your routine to find that sweet spot where you're challenging yourself but not overdoing it. For example, if you notice that your heart rate is consistently high during workouts, consider incorporating more rest days or switching to lower-intensity activities. If dehydration is an issue, set reminders to drink water at regular intervals throughout the day, not just during workouts. If your energy levels are flagging, you might need to adjust your eating window to ensure you're getting enough fuel before and after your workouts.

Monitoring your physical response to exercise while fasting is all about paying attention to the details. By keeping an eye on key indicators like heart rate, hydration status, and energy levels, and using tools and technologies to track them, you can make informed decisions about your exercise routine. Interpreting body signals helps you understand when to push harder and when to pull back, ensuring you're getting the most out of your workouts without compromising your health. Making feedback-driven adjustments based on this ongoing monitoring allows you to find the right balance between exercise and fasting, optimizing both for better overall health and well-being.

As you continue this journey of integrating intermittent fasting with physical activity, remember that each step you take is a stride toward better health and vitality. Up next, we'll explore how intermittent fasting can enhance your overall lifestyle, from better sleep to improved stress management.

HELP BUILD A SISTERHOOD OF EMPOWERED WOMEN

"Every woman's success should be an inspiration to another. We're strongest when we cheer each other on."

— SERENA WILLIAMS

You've officially made it halfway through this text and I hope that means you are busy scheduling your essential medical checks, weighing the pros and cons of each fasting window, and creating meal plans and shopping lists of healthy foods. I remember how I felt when I first started intermittent fasting and how good it felt to get the ball rolling and start taking steps toward a more energized, youthful version of myself.

One of the best things about conducting the research for this book was meeting women who had been struggling with the symptoms caused by hormonal stages, and watching them flourish. Many have commented that when they started fasting, they simply wanted relief from hot flashes, sleepless nights, and mood swings. However, they were never prepared for all the add-ons, including more balanced blood sugar levels, enhanced mental clarity, and reduced joint pain. It was also fantastic to see friends who had struggled with weight gain lose the extra five to ten pounds they had always complained about.

These women inspired me with their humor, camaraderie, and generosity. They shared delicious recipes, tips, and social media posts, all to reach other women and let them know that intermittent fasting can help make this time of life one of the most pleasantly surprising and vibrant of their lives. If you'd like to join this thriving, giving community of empowered women, why not let new readers know what you think of this book?

By leaving a review of this book on Amazon, you'll let other women over 50 know where they can find a complete guide on how to craft a personalized intermittent fasting plan that best suits their lifestyle.

Thanks for your enthusiasm. It'll take just a minute to share your opinion, but it could inspire another woman who is currently struggling with hormonal ups and downs that affect many women over 50.

Scan the QR code below

6

OVERCOMING PSYCHOLOGICAL BARRIERS

I magine you're about to start a new chapter in a book, but this one isn't just about your favorite detective solving mysteries. It's about you, taking charge of your health and well-being. The pages are blank, and you're the author of your own story. Sounds exciting, right? But also a bit intimidating? Let's be honest, the mental hurdles can sometimes feel like climbing Everest. But no worries, we're here to tackle those together.

6.1 COMMON MENTAL CHALLENGES AND HOW TO OVERCOME THEM

First, let's identify the mental roadblocks that often pop up when starting intermittent fasting. One of the most common fears is the fear of hunger. The thought of going hours without eating can send shivers down your spine, especially if you've been used to regular meals and snacks all your life. Hunger can feel like a relentless nag, but it's crucial to understand that it's often more psychological than physical. Recognize and name this barrier: "I'm afraid of being hungry." Once you've named it, you can start to address it. Another common barrier is anxiety about changing long-standing eating habits. Change can be scary, and the thought of altering your daily routine might cause some sleepless nights. Recognize this anxiety and voice it: "I'm anxious about changing my eating habits." Lastly, resistance to lifestyle change is a big one. We are creatures of habit, and breaking old patterns isn't easy. Admit this resistance: "I'm resistant to changing my lifestyle."

Now, let's tackle these barriers with cognitive restructuring techniques. This fancy term simply means changing the way you think about fasting. Instead of viewing hunger as a negative experience, reframe it as a sign that your body is working hard to improve your health. Think of it as your body cleaning house, getting rid of old, damaged cells and making way for new, healthy ones. Tell yourself, "Hunger is a sign that my body is healing and becoming more efficient." When anxiety about changing eating habits creeps in, remind yourself of the benefits. Visualize how you'll feel more energetic, less bloated, and more in control of your health. Replace thoughts like "I can't do this" with "I am capable of making positive changes for my well-being." Cognitive restructuring is about catching those negative thoughts and flipping them on their heads.

Stress management is another crucial component. Let's face it, stress can be a real party crasher, making everything feel ten times harder. Incorporate deep breathing exercises into your daily routine. When you feel overwhelmed, take a moment to breathe deeply. Inhale for four counts, hold for four counts, and exhale for four counts. This helps activate the body's relaxation response. Progressive muscle relaxation is another excellent technique. Start by tensing and then slowly relaxing each muscle group, beginning with your toes and working your way up to your head. This can help reduce physical tension and calm your mind. Guided imagery is like a mini-vacation for your brain. Close your eyes and visualize a peaceful, calming place, whether it's a beach, a forest, or your cozy living room. Imagine all the smells, sounds, and sensations of that place. This mental escape can help reduce stress and make fasting feel more manageable.

Sometimes, self-managed strategies aren't enough, and that's perfectly okay. Seeking support from mental health professionals can be incredibly beneficial, especially if you have a history of eating disorders or severe anxiety. A therapist can provide personalized strategies and support to help you navigate the psychological aspects of intermittent fasting. They can help you develop healthy coping mechanisms, challenge negative thought patterns, and provide a safe space to express your fears and concerns. Remember, seeking professional support isn't a sign of weakness; it's a proactive step towards better mental health and overall well-being.

Reflective Exercise: Naming Your Barriers

Take a few minutes to write down your biggest psychological barriers to intermittent fasting. Next to each barrier, jot down a positive reframe or strategy to overcome it. For example:

- Barrier: "I'm afraid of being hungry."
    - Reframe: "Hunger is a sign that my body is healing."
- Barrier: "I'm anxious about changing my eating habits."
    - Strategy: Visualize the benefits of fasting.

Identifying and addressing these mental challenges is the first step towards overcoming them. By recognizing your fears, reframing negative thoughts, incorporating stress management techniques, and seeking professional support when needed, you can navigate the psychological hurdles of intermittent fasting with confidence and resilience.

6.2 MAINTAINING MOTIVATION AND DEALING WITH PLATEAUS

Sticking to any new habit, especially one as life-changing as intermittent fasting, can feel like climbing a mountain. But instead of focusing only on the peak, let's talk about setting incremental goals that make the climb enjoyable and manageable. Imagine breaking down your ultimate goal into smaller, bite-sized milestones. Whether it's making it through your first 12-hour fast or hitting a week of consistent 16/8 fasting, these tiny victories add up. Write down these goals, and celebrate each one. Maybe treat yourself to a new book or a relaxing bath when you reach a milestone. These small rewards can keep you motivated and make the process feel like a series of wins rather than one daunting task.

Handling plateaus can be one of the most frustrating parts of any health regimen. You've been fasting diligently, but the scale just won't budge. First, take a deep breath. Plateaus are perfectly normal. They're your body's way of adjusting to its new routine. To break through a plateau, start by reassessing your fasting protocol. Are you sticking to your eating windows? Are you consuming nutrient-dense foods? Sometimes, a little tweak can make a big difference. Perhaps try shifting your eating window by an hour or incorporating a different fasting method like the 5:2. Another strategy is to shake up your diet within your eating window. Introduce more protein, reduce processed carbs, or add more fiber. Your body might just need a little nudge to get moving again.

Motivational affirmations can be like a secret weapon in your fasting toolkit. These are positive statements that remind you of your strength and why you started this journey in the first place.

Create personalized affirmations that resonate with you. For example, "I embrace the strength within me to fast successfully," or "My body is healing and rejuvenating through fasting." Repeat these affirmations every morning or whenever you feel your motivation waning. Write them on sticky notes and place them around your home. Seeing these positive messages throughout the day can boost your spirits and keep you focused on your goals. They serve as gentle reminders that you're capable and strong, even when the going gets tough.

Engaging with community forums or support groups can provide a wellspring of motivation. Sharing your journey with others who understand your challenges can be incredibly empowering. Online forums, social media groups, or local meet-ups can be great places to connect. These communities offer a space to share success stories, exchange tips, and celebrate milestones together. Imagine logging onto a forum and reading about someone who broke through their plateau after a month of struggle. Their success can reignite your own motivation. Plus, offering support to others can create a sense of camaraderie and shared purpose. You're not just in this for yourself; you're part of a larger community working towards better health together.

Picture Mary, a 58-year-old who felt stuck after losing 10 pounds with intermittent fasting. She joined an online fasting group and found a treasure trove of advice and encouragement. One member suggested she try the 5:2 method for a few weeks. Mary gave it a shot and saw her weight start to drop again. The support and shared experiences from the community gave her the boost she needed to keep going. Success stories like Mary's highlight the importance of community support in maintaining motivation and overcoming challenges.

By setting small, achievable goals, reassessing your approach when needed, using motivational affirmations, and engaging with supportive communities, you can maintain your motivation and handle plateaus effectively. The journey of intermittent fasting is filled with ups and downs, but with the right strategies, you can stay on track and achieve your health goals.

6.3 THE ROLE OF MINDFULNESS IN INTERMITTENT FASTING

Let's be real—sometimes, the hardest part of intermittent fasting isn't the fasting itself but managing our relationship with food. Imagine sitting down to eat and truly savoring every bite, noticing the flavors, textures, and even the emotions that come with it. This is where mindfulness can transform your eating habits. By promoting a greater awareness of hunger and satiety cues, mindfulness helps you recognize when you're genuinely hungry versus when you're eating out of habit or emotion. When you eat mindfully, you're more likely to make choices that nourish your body, rather than just filling it. It's about listening to what your body truly needs, not just what your mind craves.

Mindfulness meditation practices can be a game-changer for enhancing focus and reducing emotional reactivity, especially around hunger. Picture this: you're halfway through your fasting period, and suddenly, the urge to snack hits you like a tidal wave. Instead of immediately reaching for something to eat, take a moment to sit quietly and focus on your breath. Inhale deeply, hold for a few seconds, and then exhale slowly. Repeat this a few times. This simple practice can help calm your mind and give you the space to decide whether you're truly hungry or just experiencing a fleeting craving. Another helpful practice is body scanning. Close your eyes and mentally scan your body from head to toe, noticing any areas of tension or discomfort. This can help you become more attuned to how your body feels and whether it really needs food or just a break.

Integrating mindfulness into your daily routine doesn't have to be complicated. Start your day with a few minutes of mindful breathing before you even get out of bed. This sets a calm tone for the day ahead. Throughout the day, take short mindfulness breaks. Whether you're waiting in line, sitting in traffic, or taking a walk, these moments of mindfulness can help you stay centered and reduce stress. When it comes to meals, make it a point to turn off distractions like the TV or your phone. Focus solely on your food. Notice the colors, smells, and textures. Take smaller bites and chew thoroughly. This not only enhances your eating experience but also helps you recognize when you're full, preventing overeating.

The broader benefits of mindfulness for mental health are profound, especially when you're dealing with the mental challenges of intermittent fasting. Mindfulness reduces anxiety by helping you stay in the present moment rather than worrying about the future or dwelling on the past. This can be particularly helpful during fasting periods when you might feel anxious about hunger or the next meal. Improved emotional regulation is another significant benefit. Mindfulness helps you respond to emotions thoughtfully rather than react impulsively. This means that when you feel a wave of hunger or a craving, you can acknowledge it without immediately giving in. Over time, this practice can strengthen your willpower and make fasting feel more manageable.

Consider using mindfulness as a tool to support your intermittent fasting practice. When you combine mindfulness with fasting, you're not just changing your eating schedule; you're transforming your relationship with food and your body. It's about creating a more intentional, aware, and compassionate approach to eating and self-care. This shift can lead to a greater sense of well-being, making intermittent fasting not just a diet but a holistic lifestyle change.

6.4 BUILDING RESILIENCE AGAINST SOCIAL AND EMOTIONAL TRIGGERS

Picture this: you're at a family gathering, and Aunt Susan is eyeing your plate, wondering why you're not diving into the mashed potatoes like you used to. Social gatherings can be a minefield for anyone trying to maintain a fasting regimen. Identifying specific triggers is the first step in building resilience. Social events, emotional stressors, or even a lack of support from friends and family can disrupt your fasting plans. It's crucial to recognize these triggers. Maybe it's the pressure to eat at a dinner party, the stress of a busy workday, or the well-meaning but persistent questions from friends. By naming these triggers, you can start to develop strategies to handle them.

Imagine having a toolkit of coping strategies to pull from when social pressures arise. One effective approach is to prepare responses to common questions or criticisms about fasting. If someone asks why you're not eating, you could say, "I'm trying out a new eating schedule for my health." Keep it simple and positive. Another strategy is to strategically share meals during social events. Plan your eating window around the event so you can enjoy the meal without feeling like you're breaking your fast. If that's not possible, focus on the social aspects rather than the food. Engage in conversations, enjoy the company, and remind yourself that it's okay to say no to food.

Building emotional resilience is like strengthening a muscle—it takes practice and patience. Journaling can be an incredibly effective technique for processing feelings and gaining insight into your emotional triggers. Write down what you're feeling and why. Are you stressed because of work? Feeling pressured by friends? Putting your thoughts on paper can help you understand and manage your emotions better. Practicing self-compassion is another vital technique. Be kind to yourself. If you slip up, don't beat yourself up. Instead, acknowledge what happened, understand why, and move on. Setting boundaries around discussions of diet and body weight can also protect your emotional well-being. If someone keeps pushing about your fasting, it's okay to say, "I'd rather not discuss my eating habits. Let's talk about something else."

Supportive relationships play a crucial role in maintaining your fasting regimen. It's important to cultivate relationships that respect your choices. Communicate your needs and boundaries clearly. Let your friends and family know why you're fasting and how they can support you. For instance, you might say, "I'm fasting to improve my health, and it would mean a lot if you could support me by not offering me food outside my eating window." If someone continues to disregard your boundaries, it might be necessary to limit your interactions with them or address the issue directly. Surrounding yourself with supportive people can make a world of difference.

Consider creating a support network of like-minded individuals. This could be a fasting group, an online forum, or even a few friends who share similar health goals. These people can offer encouragement, share tips, and celebrate your successes with you. Imagine having a friend who understands exactly what you're going through and can offer a pep talk when you're feeling low. These relationships can provide a sense of community and shared purpose, making the fasting experience more enjoyable and less isolating.

By identifying specific social and emotional triggers, developing coping strategies, building emotional resilience, and cultivating supportive relationships, you can maintain your fasting regimen with confidence and ease. Remember, it's not about being perfect, but about finding what works for you and making adjustments as needed.

6.5 CELEBRATING MILESTONES AND NON-SCALE VICTORIES

When you think about progress, it's natural to picture the numbers on the scale moving in the right direction. But let's broaden that view a bit. Non-scale victories are just as important, if not more so. Have you noticed your energy levels soaring, like you've had an extra shot of espresso without actually drinking one? Or maybe you're sleeping better, waking up refreshed and ready to tackle the day. These improvements are huge wins. Enhanced mental clarity is another fantastic non-scale victory. That fog lifting from your brain? That's worth celebrating. And let's not forget the feelings of empowerment you get from sticking to your fasting plan. These victories might not show up on the scale, but they're monumental in your overall well-being.

Creating a reward system can make these milestones feel even more special. Think about the last time you accomplished something significant. How did you celebrate? Now, apply that to your fasting achievements. Each milestone deserves recognition. For instance, if you've successfully completed a week of your new fasting schedule, treat yourself to a new book you've been eyeing. Hit the one-month mark? Maybe it's time for a day out at the spa or a new outfit. The key is to make these rewards non-food related, so you're not undermining your progress. Rewards can be simple pleasures like a relaxing day out, a new piece of jewelry, or even a movie night. These treats give you something to look forward to and make the entire process more enjoyable.

Reflective practices are another powerful way to acknowledge and celebrate your progress. Keeping a progress journal can be incredibly rewarding. Each day, take a few minutes to jot down how you're feeling, any challenges you faced, and the victories you achieved. Reflect on your journey, no matter how small the steps may seem. Over time, you'll see how far you've come. This journal can serve as a reminder of your growth and resilience. On those tough days when motivation wanes, looking back at your progress can reignite your determination. It's a tangible way to see your hard work paying off, and it helps you stay focused on your long-term goals.

Sharing achievements with others can also be a fantastic motivator. Whether it's with a support group, friends, or social media, sharing your milestones can provide external validation and boost your confidence. Imagine the joy of posting about your improved sleep quality or increased energy levels and receiving encouraging comments from others who understand your journey. This external support can be incredibly motivating. It's like having your own cheerleading squad, rooting for your success. Plus, sharing your story might inspire others to start their own fasting journey, creating a ripple effect of positive change.

Let's talk about Jane, a 55-year-old woman who decided to try intermittent fasting to improve her health. She started with small goals, like completing a 12-hour fast. Each time she hit a milestone, she rewarded herself with a non-food treat, like a new book or a relaxing day out. Jane also kept a progress journal, documenting her improved energy levels, better sleep, and enhanced mental clarity. She shared these achievements with her support group and received overwhelming encouragement. This validation boosted her confidence and kept her motivated to continue. Jane's story highlights the importance of celebrating non-scale victories and sharing achievements with others.

Celebrating milestones and non-scale victories is about recognizing the whole picture of your health and well-being. It's not just about the numbers on the scale but about how you feel, how you sleep, and how empowered you are. By creating a reward system, engaging in reflective practices, and sharing your achievements, you can stay motivated and enjoy the journey of intermittent fasting. Take a moment to celebrate each step, no matter how small, and cherish the progress you're making towards a healthier, happier you.

In the next chapter, we'll explore how intermittent fasting can become a part of your holistic health journey. From improving sleep quality to managing stress, we'll dive into the broader benefits that make intermittent fasting a sustainable and rewarding lifestyle choice.

7

FASTING AS A PART OF HOLISTIC HEALTH

Picture this: It's 3 AM, and you're wide awake, staring at the ceiling, counting sheep, and wondering why sleep is playing hard to get. The nights are long, and the days are groggy. Sound familiar? You're not alone. Many women over 50 find sleep elusive, and the struggle is real. The good news? Intermittent fasting might just be the magic key to unlock those sweet dreams.

7.1 ENHANCING SLEEP QUALITY THROUGH FASTING

Understanding how intermittent fasting can improve sleep quality starts with a peek into our body's natural rhythms. Our bodies operate on a circadian rhythm—a 24-hour internal clock that regulates sleep and wakefulness. This rhythm is influenced by various factors, including light exposure and, you guessed it, meal times. Intermittent fasting helps align these meal times with your body's natural cycles, which can lead to better sleep. When you eat during a set window and fast the rest of the time, your body starts to anticipate these periods, creating a predictable routine that supports your circadian rhythm. Imagine your body as an orchestra, with each instrument playing in perfect harmony. That's what intermittent fasting can do for your circadian rhythm.

Practical tips for optimizing sleep while fasting are surprisingly straightforward. First, try to time your eating window so that you avoid heavy meals close to bedtime. A full stomach can make it harder to fall asleep and stay asleep. Instead, aim to finish your last meal at least three hours before hitting the hay. This gives your body ample time to digest, reducing the likelihood of discomfort that can keep you tossing and turning. Also, minimize caffeine intake during the latter part of the day. While that afternoon coffee might seem like a lifesaver, it can sabotage your sleep later. Opt for herbal teas or water instead. Creating a bedtime routine that signals your body it's time to wind down—like reading a book or taking a warm bath—can also work wonders.

The impact of improved sleep extends far beyond just feeling more rested. Better sleep leads to better hormonal balance. When you sleep well, your body regulates cortisol (the stress hormone) more effectively, which can help reduce overall stress levels. Improved mood is another perk. A good night's sleep can make you feel like you can conquer the world, or at least the day ahead. And let's not forget cognitive function. Quality sleep enhances memory, decision-making skills, and overall brain health. It's like giving your brain a mini-vacation every night, allowing it to recharge and perform at its best.

Addressing potential sleep disturbances during intermittent fasting is crucial for success. You might initially experience difficulty falling asleep due to hunger or changes in energy levels. If hunger is keeping you awake, consider adjusting your eating window slightly or incorporating more protein and fiber into your last meal to keep you satiated longer. Sometimes, a small, nutrient-dense snack like a handful of almonds can help. If changes in energy levels are the culprit, try incorporating relaxation techniques before bed, such as deep breathing exercises or meditation. These practices can help calm your mind and prepare your body for restful sleep.

Let's do a quick exercise to help you fine-tune your sleep routine.

Sleep Optimization Checklist

1. **Finish Eating:** Complete your last meal at least three hours before bedtime.
2. **Limit Caffeine:** Avoid caffeine after 2 PM.
3. **Create a Routine:** Develop a bedtime routine (reading, warm bath, meditation).
4. **Adjust Diet:** Ensure your last meal includes protein and fiber.
5. **Relaxation Techniques:** Practice deep breathing or meditation before bed.

Following this checklist can help you harness the full benefits of intermittent fasting, ensuring that you not only sleep better, but also wake up feeling refreshed and ready to tackle whatever the day throws your way.

7.2 STRESS REDUCTION TECHNIQUES COMPATIBLE WITH INTERMITTENT FASTING

Imagine you've just started intermittent fasting, and suddenly, your stress levels seem to spike. You're not imagining things. Changes in diet and routine can initially increase stress levels. Your body, used to a certain eating schedule, is now adjusting to a new rhythm. This transitional phase can be challenging but manageable with the right strategies. Begin by acknowledging that it's normal to feel a bit off-kilter at first. Your body is learning to adapt, and this takes time. A great way to manage this transition is to start slowly. Instead of jumping into a 16/8 schedule right away, try shorter fasting windows and gradually lengthen them as your body adjusts.

Stress-reduction techniques can be lifesavers during these periods. Guided meditations are a wonderful way to center yourself. Apps like Calm or Headspace offer short, guided sessions that can fit into any schedule. Picture this: you're feeling the afternoon slump and the stress creeping in. Take ten minutes to listen to a soothing voice guide you through a meditation. It's like hitting a mental reset button. Breathing exercises are another effective tool. Try the 4-7-8 technique: inhale for four seconds, hold for seven, and exhale for eight. This simple practice can calm your nervous system and reduce stress almost instantly. Gentle yoga is also a fantastic way to relax. Focus on poses that emphasize stretching and deep breathing, like Child's Pose or Cat-Cow. Even five minutes on the mat can make a big difference.

Incorporating these practices into your daily routine can provide ongoing support. Carve out specific times in your day dedicated to stress reduction. Maybe it's ten minutes of meditation after lunch or a gentle yoga session before bed. The key is consistency. Just like fasting, these techniques work best when they become a regular part of your life. Consider creating a stress-reduction toolkit. Fill it with things that make you feel good—a favorite book, a playlist of calming music, or even a small journal for jotting down thoughts. Having these items readily available can make it easier to turn to them when stress levels rise.

Monitoring your stress levels is crucial for making necessary adjustments. Pay attention to how you feel throughout the day. Are you more irritable than usual? Do you feel overwhelmed or anxious? These can be signs that your stress levels are creeping up. Consider keeping a stress diary. Note down when you feel stressed, what triggered it, and how you responded. This can help you identify patterns and make informed adjustments to your fasting routine or stress management strategies. If you notice persistent high stress, it might be time to tweak your fasting window or incorporate more relaxation techniques into your day.

Here's a simple exercise to help monitor your stress levels effectively:

Stress Monitoring Checklist

1. **Daily Log:** Keep a daily log of your stress levels on a scale from 1-10.
2. **Identify Triggers:** Note what triggers your stress (e.g., work, hunger, social interactions).
3. **Response Tracking:** Record how you responded to stress (e.g., meditation, breathing exercises, yoga).
4. **Weekly Review:** Review your log at the end of each week to identify patterns and necessary adjustments.

By integrating stress-reduction techniques into your daily routine and monitoring your stress levels, you can create a supportive environment that enhances your intermittent fasting experience. Remember, the goal is not just to manage stress but to build resilience, making it easier to stick to your fasting schedule and reap its full benefits.

7.3 THE IMPACT OF FASTING ON EMOTIONAL WELL-BEING

Imagine waking up each day feeling a bit lighter, not just in body but in spirit. Intermittent fasting doesn't just trim the waistline; it also offers a boost to your emotional well-being. One of the most profound emotional benefits of fasting is the sense of empower-ment it brings. When you successfully adhere to a fasting sched-ule, it feels like a personal victory. This accomplishment can significantly improve self-esteem, making you feel more in control of your health and your life. The consistent structure of intermit-tent fasting can instill a sense of discipline that spills over into other areas, making you feel capable and strong. It's like winning a small battle every day, and who doesn't love a victory?

Navigating the emotional challenges that come with intermittent fasting is an important skill. It's normal to feel frustrated or impa-tient, especially when progress seems slow. Cognitive reframing can be a valuable tool here. Instead of viewing a slow week as a failure, see it as a period of adjustment. Your body is recalibrat-ing, and that's a good thing. Journaling can also help. Write down your thoughts and feelings about your fasting experience. Are you feeling irritable? Note it. Did you resist the urge to snack? Celebrate that win in your journal. This practice can help you process emotions constructively and keep you motivated.

Enhancing emotional awareness during fasting is another layer of this journey. Mindful eating is a practice worth adopting. Instead of eating mindlessly while scrolling through social media, take a moment to truly savor your food. Notice the textures, flavors, and aromas. This not only enhances your eating experience but also helps you become more attuned to your body's hunger and full-ness cues. Self-reflection is equally important. Take time to ponder how your relationship with food has evolved. Are you eating out of hunger, boredom, or emotion? Understanding these triggers can help you develop healthier habits and a more balanced relationship with food.

Sustained intermittent fasting can contribute to long-term emotional health improvements. Over time, the discipline and structure of fasting can foster emotional resilience. You'll find that you're better equipped to handle life's ups and downs. The sense of accomplishment from sticking to your fasting plan can boost your overall mood and make you feel more balanced. This emotional stability can lead to a more fulfilling lifestyle, where you feel in control and capable of achieving your health goals.

Intermittent fasting is more than just a dietary regimen; it's a holistic approach that can transform your emotional well-being. By embracing the emotional benefits, navigating challenges with cognitive reframing and journaling, enhancing emotional awareness through mindful eating, and fostering long-term emotional health, you can create a balanced and fulfilling lifestyle.

7.4 ANTI-AGING EFFECTS OF INTERMITTENT FASTING

Imagine a world where you can slow down the aging clock. It's not science fiction—intermittent fasting offers cellular and molecular benefits that can make this a reality. One of the key mechanisms at play is autophagy, a process where your body cleans out damaged cells and regenerates new ones. Think of it as your body's housekeeping service, tidying up cellular debris and making room for fresh, healthy cells. This enhanced autophagy helps reduce inflammation, which is a major contributor to aging and many chronic diseases. Moreover, intermittent fasting improves DNA repair mechanisms, essentially patching up the wear and tear that accumulates over time. It's like having a built-in repair crew working around the clock to keep you in tip-top shape.

When it comes to visible signs of aging, intermittent fasting doesn't disappoint. Many women over 50 report improvements in skin health, including a reduction in age spots and a more youthful appearance. How, you ask? By promoting cellular health and reducing inflammation, fasting helps your skin retain its elasticity and glow. It's like giving your skin a rejuvenating spa treatment from the inside out. The reduction in oxidative stress, thanks to the improved balance of antioxidants and free radicals, also plays a crucial role. You might notice that your skin feels firmer, looks more radiant, and even those pesky wrinkles seem to soften. It's the kind of transformation that makes you want to skip the makeup and show off your natural beauty.

But the benefits don't stop at skin deep. Intermittent fasting has profound cognitive and neurological effects that contribute to anti-aging. Studies have shown that fasting can enhance brain function by promoting neurogenesis, the growth of new neurons. This improves memory, learning, and overall cognitive function. The increase in brain-derived neurotrophic factor (BDNF) supports neuron survival and growth, making your brain more resilient to stress and aging. Additionally, intermittent fasting can lower the risk of neurodegenerative diseases like Alzheimer's and Parkinson's by reducing neuroinflammation. It's like giving your brain a protective shield that keeps it sharp and focused, even as the years go by.

To complement the anti-aging effects of intermittent fasting, incorporating specific foods and supplements into your diet can amplify the benefits. Antioxidant-rich foods like berries, dark chocolate, and green tea help neutralize free radicals, reducing oxidative stress and promoting cellular health. Omega-3 fatty acids, found in fatty fish like salmon, flaxseeds, and walnuts, support brain health and reduce inflammation. Consider adding a quality multivitamin to ensure you're getting all the essential nutrients, especially if your diet has gaps. These anti-aging foods and supplements work in harmony with your fasting routine, enhancing the overall impact on your longevity and well-being.

So, picture this: you're enjoying a delicious salmon salad sprinkled with walnuts and a side of mixed berries. Not only are you treating your taste buds, but you're also fueling your body with powerful anti-aging nutrients. It's a win-win that makes sticking to your fasting schedule even more rewarding. And the best part? You don't need to overhaul your entire diet. Small, consistent changes can make a big difference. Maybe start with adding a handful of berries to your breakfast or swapping out a snack for a piece of dark chocolate. Over time, these little adjustments can add up to significant anti-aging benefits, both inside and out.

7.5 FASTING FOR LONGEVITY AND DISEASE PREVENTION

Imagine a life where you feel vibrant, energetic, and disease-free well into your golden years. Research shows that intermittent fasting can help make this a reality by extending lifespan and reducing the risk of age-related diseases. Studies have linked intermittent fasting to a decreased incidence of cardiovascular disease, diabetes, and even cancer. For example, a review published in the New England Journal of Medicine highlighted how fasting triggers a metabolic switch from glucose-based to ketone-based energy, which enhances stress resistance and longevity. This metabolic switch is not just about burning fat; it's about optimizing your body's overall function for a longer, healthier life.

The mechanisms by which intermittent fasting prevents disease are fascinating. Improved metabolic health is one of the key benefits. Fasting helps regulate blood sugar levels and increases insulin sensitivity, reducing the risk of type 2 diabetes. Enhanced immune function is another crucial factor. When you fast, your body initiates autophagy, a process that removes damaged cells and regenerates new ones, boosting your immune system's efficiency. Hormonal balance also plays a significant role. Fasting helps regulate hormones like insulin, ghrelin (the hunger hormone), and leptin (the satiety hormone), creating a harmonious internal environment that supports overall health. These mechanisms work together to create a robust defense against chronic diseases, making you feel like you've discovered the secret to eternal youth.

Personalizing your intermittent fasting approach to suit individual health conditions can maximize disease prevention benefits while ensuring safety. If you have a specific health condition like diabetes, it's vital to consult with your healthcare provider to tailor your fasting plan. For instance, shorter fasting windows might be more appropriate, or you may need to monitor your blood sugar levels more frequently. If you're dealing with hypertension, incorporating potassium-rich foods during your eating window can help manage blood pressure. The goal is to create a fasting regimen that aligns with your unique health needs, ensuring that you reap the benefits without compromising your well-being.

Integrating intermittent fasting into a lifestyle focused on longevity and disease prevention can be both seamless and rewarding. Regular physical activity is a cornerstone of this approach. Aim for a mix of aerobic exercises and strength training to keep your body strong and agile. Mental health practices like mindfulness and meditation can complement fasting by reducing stress and promoting emotional well-being. Community engagement is equally important. Surround yourself with a supportive network of friends, or join groups that share your health goals. This sense of community can provide motivation, encouragement, and a sense of belonging, making it easier to stick to your fasting routine.

Imagine starting your day with a brisk walk in the park, followed by a nutritious meal within your eating window. As the day progresses, you engage in activities that stimulate your mind and soul, whether it's a yoga class, a book club meeting, or a hobby you love. By evening, you enjoy a light, balanced meal and wind down with some relaxation techniques before bed. This holistic approach not only supports intermittent fasting but also fosters a lifestyle that promotes longevity and disease prevention.

With these practices in place, you'll find that intermittent fasting becomes a natural part of your day, contributing to a longer, healthier, and more fulfilling life.

7.6 FASTING AND ITS EFFECTS ON BRAIN HEALTH

Picture this: you've just walked into a room and actually remember why you're there. No more standing in front of the fridge, wondering what you came for! Intermittent fasting has some incredible neuroprotective effects that can help keep your brain sharp and your memory intact. One of the key players here is something called brain-derived neurotrophic factor (BDNF). This protein supports the growth and protection of neurons, the cells in your brain that transmit information. Increased production of BDNF, often triggered by fasting, acts like a fertilizer for your brain cells, encouraging growth and repair. This boost in BDNF can potentially reduce the risk of neurodegenerative diseases like Alzheimer's and Parkinson's. Imagine it as a protective bubble wrapping around your neurons, keeping them safe and sound.

But the benefits don't stop at growth and protection. Intermittent fasting can also enhance brain function in remarkable ways. Studies have shown that fasting improves cognitive functions such as memory, learning, and even problem-solving skills. How does this happen? It's all about mitochondrial function. Mitochondria are the powerhouses of your cells, providing the energy needed for cellular activities. When you fast, your mitochondria become more efficient, producing energy more effectively and reducing the production of harmful free radicals. This improved mitochondrial function means your brain cells have more energy to perform their tasks, leading to better cognitive performance. It's like upgrading your brain's operating system to the latest, most efficient version.

Another fascinating aspect of intermittent fasting is its impact on neuroinflammation. Neuroinflammation is an inflammatory response within the brain and is a common factor in many degenerative brain diseases. Fasting helps to moderate the levels of inflammatory cytokines, the proteins that promote inflammation. By reducing these cytokines, fasting can lower neuroinflammation, thus protecting your brain from the damaging effects of chronic inflammation. Think of it as putting out a smoldering fire before it turns into a full-blown blaze. This reduction in inflammation not only protects your brain cells but also enhances overall brain health, making your mind clearer and more focused.

The long-term benefits of consistent intermittent fasting on brain health are truly impressive. Research suggests that regular fasting can contribute to the delay or even prevention of neurodegenerative diseases. By maintaining the production of neurotrophic factors like BDNF, improving mitochondrial efficiency, and reducing neuroinflammation, fasting creates an environment where your brain cells can thrive. This means that as you age, you're more likely to retain your cognitive abilities, stay mentally agile, and enjoy a better quality of life. It's like having a long-term insurance policy for your brain, one that pays dividends in the form of mental clarity and resilience.

Incorporating intermittent fasting into your lifestyle can seem daunting, but the cognitive and neurological benefits make it well worth the effort. Imagine being able to recall names, dates, and where you left your keys with ease. Picture yourself engaging in conversations, solving puzzles, and navigating daily tasks with a sharp and agile mind. The science behind intermittent fasting and brain health is compelling, offering a natural and effective way to maintain and even enhance your mental faculties as you age. So, as you continue your fasting journey, remember that you're not just investing in your physical health but also in the long-term vitality of your brain.

8

ADVANCED STRATEGIES AND TROUBLESHOOTING

Picture this: you're at a family gathering, and Aunt Sue, who's never held back an opinion in her life, corners you in the kitchen. "So, what's this fasting thing you're doing? Isn't it bad for your hormones?" she asks, eyebrow raised. You take a deep breath, ready to defend your choices, but wouldn't it be great to have all the answers? Let's dive into fine-tuning your fasting for optimal hormonal balance, so next time Aunt Sue corners you, you'll be armed with knowledge and confidence.

8.1 FINE-TUNING YOUR FASTING FOR HORMONAL BALANCE

Hormonal imbalances can feel like you're living with a mischievous gremlin that's wreaking havoc on your body. Symptoms might include irregular periods (if you're still in that stage), sleep disturbances where you feel like you're starring in your own insomnia marathon, or unexpected weight gain that seems to appear out of nowhere. These symptoms can be both a cause and an effect of fasting, making it essential to navigate this terrain with care.

Adjusting your fasting windows can be a game-changer. If you find yourself waking up at 3 AM, unable to fall back to sleep, it might be worth experimenting with the timing of your fasting periods. Some studies suggest that consuming food earlier in the day can have beneficial effects on hormones. For instance, if you typically fast from 8 PM to noon the next day, try shifting your window to 6 PM to 10 AM. This slight adjustment can help stabilize your cortisol levels, the pesky stress hormone that loves to spike just when you're trying to relax. Alternatively, if you notice that your energy levels dip significantly during the day, consider shortening your fasting period. Perhaps a 14/10 schedule (14 hours of fasting and a 10-hour eating window) might be more sustainable for you.

Dietary adjustments also play a crucial role in supporting hormonal balance. Including hormone-supportive foods during your eating windows can make a significant difference. Phytoestrogen-rich foods, such as flaxseeds, soy products, and legumes, can help balance estrogen levels. These foods mimic estrogen in the body and can be particularly beneficial for women experiencing a decline in estrogen due to menopause. Additionally, incorporating healthy fats like avocado, nuts, and olive oil can support overall hormone production. Omega-3 fatty acids, found in fatty fish like salmon and mackerel, are also excellent for reducing inflammation and supporting hormone health.

Monitoring and adjusting based on feedback is vital. Your body is incredibly adept at giving you clues about what it needs—you just have to listen. Keep a journal to track your symptoms and how they correlate with your fasting and eating patterns. Note any changes in your sleep quality, mood, energy levels, and menstrual cycle if applicable. This data can be incredibly insightful. For instance, if you notice that your sleep improves when you eat your last meal earlier, stick with that. If you find that certain foods exacerbate your symptoms, consider eliminating them for a period to see if there's a noticeable difference.

Consulting with a healthcare provider can provide personalized guidance. They can help interpret your symptoms in the context of your overall health and make recommendations that align with your specific needs. For example, if you're experiencing significant sleep disturbances, they might suggest checking your melatonin levels or exploring other underlying causes. They can also help you fine-tune your fasting schedule and dietary choices to support your hormonal health optimally.

Hormonal Balance Checklist

1. **Track Symptoms:** Keep a daily journal of sleep patterns, mood, energy levels, and menstrual cycle changes.
2. **Adjust Fasting Windows:** Experiment with different fasting periods to see what works best for your body.
3. **Include Hormone-Supportive Foods:** Add flaxseeds, soy, legumes, healthy fats, and Omega-3 rich foods to your diet.
4. **Monitor and Adapt:** Regularly review your journal and make necessary adjustments to your fasting and eating patterns.
5. **Consult Healthcare Providers:** Seek personalized advice to address specific hormonal imbalances and overall health needs.

By fine-tuning your fasting routine to support hormonal balance, you can navigate the complexities of menopause with greater ease and confidence. Next time Aunt Sue has questions, you'll not only have the answers, but also the results to back them up.

8.2 DEALING WITH UNEXPECTED SIDE EFFECTS

You wake up one morning, excited to tackle the day, only to be greeted by a pounding headache. Or perhaps you stand up too quickly and feel a wave of dizziness wash over you. These are just a couple of the common side effects that can make intermittent fasting feel like a bit of a rollercoaster. But don't worry, you're not alone, and there are ways to navigate these bumps in the road.

Headaches are a common complaint when starting intermittent fasting. They often occur because your body is adjusting to a new rhythm that includes longer periods without food. Dehydration can also be a culprit since you're not getting as much water from food. To combat this, make sure to drink plenty of water throughout the day. Herbal teas and infused water with a splash of lemon or cucumber can make staying hydrated more enjoyable. If the headache persists, consider a small snack like a handful of nuts or a piece of fruit to see if that helps.

Dizziness is another side effect that can make you feel like you've just stepped off a merry-go-round. This often happens because your blood sugar levels are adjusting to the new fasting schedule. To address dizziness, ensure you're consuming balanced meals during your eating windows that include a mix of protein, healthy fats, and complex carbohydrates. These nutrients help stabilize blood sugar levels and keep you feeling steady. If dizziness continues, take it as a cue to shorten your fasting window until your body adjusts.

Constipation can also rear its unwelcome head. This can happen because fasting changes your eating patterns, which can affect your digestive system. To keep things moving smoothly, increase your fiber intake by eating more fruits, vegetables, and whole grains during your eating window. Drinking plenty of water also helps, as does regular physical activity. A gentle walk after meals can be particularly effective in aiding digestion and preventing constipation.

Sometimes, these side effects can be more than just minor inconveniences. It's important to know when to seek medical advice. If your headaches are severe and persistent despite staying hydrated and adjusting your diet, it might be time to consult a healthcare provider. The same goes for dizziness that doesn't improve with dietary adjustments or if you feel faint. Constipation that lasts for more than a few days despite increasing fiber and water intake should also be discussed with a healthcare professional. They can help rule out any underlying conditions and provide guidance tailored to your specific needs.

Preventing these side effects often comes down to understanding their causes and making proactive adjustments. For instance, if you know that dehydration can lead to headaches, make a habit of carrying a water bottle with you and sipping throughout the day. If blood sugar dips cause dizziness, planning balanced meals that include a mix of macronutrients can help. For constipation, incorporating high-fiber foods and regular physical activity into your routine can make a big difference. Monitoring your body's responses and making small tweaks to your fasting schedule and dietary choices can prevent these side effects from becoming ongoing issues.

8.3 WHEN AND HOW TO BREAK A FAST SAFELY

Imagine you're nearing the end of a 16-hour fast, and your stomach starts growling like a bear that just woke up from hibernation. It's tempting to dive into a big meal, but breaking a fast safely is crucial to maintaining your well-being. Signs that it's time to break a fast can include significant fatigue, mental fog, or severe hunger pangs. These signals indicate that your body needs nourishment, and ignoring them can lead to overeating later.

When it's time to end your fast, start gently. Opt for light, easily digestible foods to avoid overwhelming your digestive system. Think of things like a small bowl of soup, a smoothie with spinach and banana, or a salad with lean protein. These choices provide essential nutrients without causing digestive distress. Eating slowly and mindfully can also help; savor each bite and listen to your body's cues for fullness.

Post-fast monitoring is key to learning from your experience and adjusting future fasting practices. Pay attention to how your body responds after breaking the fast. Do you feel energized or sluggish? Are there any digestive issues? Keeping a journal to note these observations can provide valuable insights. This information can guide adjustments to your fasting schedule or dietary choices, ensuring that future fasts are more comfortable and effective.

Handling overeating post-fast requires a bit of strategy. Pre-planning your post-fast meal can make a big difference. Choose foods that are satisfying yet moderate in portion size. For example, a small portion of grilled chicken with a side of vegetables can be both nourishing and filling. Avoid high-carb or sugary foods that can cause rapid glucose spikes and leave you feeling tired and hungry soon after. Instead, focus on low-glycemic index foods that provide sustained energy.

By breaking your fast with care and monitoring your body's responses, you can maintain the benefits of intermittent fasting while minimizing any potential downsides.

8.4 WHEN AND HOW TO BREAK A FAST SAFELY

You're nearing the end of your fasting window, and suddenly, you feel a wave of fatigue that makes you want to crawl back into bed. Or maybe it's a mental fog that makes you forget why you walked into a room. These are your body's not-so-subtle hints that it might be time to break your fast. Significant fatigue, mental fog, or severe hunger pangs are all signs that your body needs nourishment. Ignoring these cues can lead to more problems down the road, like irritability or even a binge-eating session later. It's important to listen to your body and know when to give it the fuel it needs.

When you're ready to end your fast, think of it as gently waking up a sleeping baby—you wouldn't want to jolt them awake with loud noises, right? The same goes for your digestive system. Safe methods to end a fast involve gradually reintroducing foods that are easy on the stomach. Start with light, easily digestible foods to avoid gastrointestinal distress. A small bowl of soup, a smoothie with some greens and a banana, or a salad with lean protein like chicken or tofu are excellent choices. These options provide essential nutrients without overwhelming your digestive system, allowing it to ease back into its job.

Once you've broken your fast, monitoring your body's response is crucial. Pay close attention to how you feel after eating. Do you feel energized or sluggish? Are there any digestive issues like bloating or discomfort? Keeping a journal can be incredibly helpful here. Note down what you ate, how you felt immediately after, and any longer-term effects you noticed. This information can guide you in adjusting your future fasting practices. For example, if you feel great after breaking your fast with a smoothie but sluggish after a heavier meal, you'll know what works best for you.

Handling overeating post-fast can be a bit tricky, especially when you're really hungry. It's tempting to dive into a big meal, but this can lead to discomfort and negate some of the benefits of fasting. One effective strategy is to pre-plan your post-fast meals so you're not making decisions when you're ravenous. Choose meals that are satisfying yet moderate in portion size. Think of a small portion of grilled salmon with a side of steamed vegetables, or a quinoa salad with mixed greens and a light vinaigrette. These meals are nutrient-dense and filling without being heavy.

Eating slowly and mindfully can also help prevent overeating. Take the time to savor each bite, chew thoroughly, and listen to your body's cues for fullness. It's easy to overeat when you're not paying attention, but by slowing down, you give your body time to signal when it's had enough. Additionally, avoid high-carb or sugary foods that can cause rapid glucose spikes, leaving you feeling tired and hungry soon after. Instead, focus on low-glycemic index foods that provide sustained energy and keep you feeling fuller longer.

Sometimes, breaking a fast might not go as smoothly as planned. You might find that certain foods don't sit well with you or that you feel hungrier than usual. This is where post-fast monitoring comes in handy. If you notice that certain foods cause discomfort, consider eliminating them for a period to see if there's a noticeable difference. If you're consistently feeling overly hungry post-fast, you might need to adjust your fasting window or the types of foods you're eating during your eating period. Consulting with a healthcare provider can also provide personalized guidance tailored to your specific needs.

Breaking a fast safely and effectively involves understanding your body's signals, choosing the right foods, and monitoring your body's response. By paying attention to these details and making small adjustments, you can ensure that your fasting experience is both beneficial and sustainable.

8.5 FASTING DURING ILLNESS OR STRESS

Imagine this: you've been rocking your intermittent fasting routine, feeling like a wellness warrior, and then—bam!—you come down with a cold. Suddenly, the thought of fasting seems as appealing as a root canal. When you're ill, your body needs all the support it can get to fight off whatever bug has decided to crash your party. Adjusting your fasting practices during illness is not just wise; it's necessary. Start by listening to your body. If you're feeling particularly rundown, it might be best to pause your fasting regimen altogether to allow your body to focus on recovery. This doesn't mean you've failed; it means you're smart enough to prioritize your health.

If you decide to continue fasting but feel under the weather, consider shortening your fasting periods. Instead of a 16-hour fast, try a 12-hour fast. This gives your body more opportunities to get the nutrients it needs to heal. Hydration is crucial here. Drink plenty of fluids like water, herbal teas, and broths to stay hydrated and support your immune system. Also, focus on nutrient-dense foods during your eating windows. Think of foods rich in vitamins and minerals, like fruits, vegetables, and lean proteins, which can give your immune system the boost it needs.

Now, let's talk about managing fasting during stressful periods. We all know life can throw curveballs—work deadlines, family issues, or just those days when everything seems to go wrong. During these times, the additional stress of fasting might feel like too much. One way to manage this is by reducing the duration or frequency of your fasts. Instead of fasting every day, try fasting every other day or reducing your fasting window from 16 hours to 10. This can help reduce the physical stress on your body, allowing you to better cope with external stressors.

Balancing emotional and physical health considerations is crucial during these challenging times. Stress affects everyone differently, and what works for one person might not work for another. Pay attention to how your body and mind are reacting to both the stress and the fasting. If you find yourself feeling overly anxious or physically drained, it might be time to ease up on the fasting. This doesn't mean abandoning it altogether but adjusting it to better suit your current state of well-being. Sometimes, a lighter approach can make all the difference, allowing you to maintain some of the benefits of fasting without adding to your stress levels.

Consultation with health professionals can provide invaluable guidance during these periods. If you're dealing with an illness or significant stress, a healthcare provider can help tailor your fasting practices to meet your individual needs. They can offer advice on what adjustments to make and how to ensure you're still getting the nutrients and support your body needs. For example, if you're taking medication that requires food, your healthcare provider can help you plan your fasting and eating windows around your medication schedule. They can also monitor your overall health to ensure that fasting is not exacerbating any existing conditions.

Imagine you're navigating a particularly stressful period at work. Deadlines are looming, and your stress levels are through the roof. In such times, reducing the fasting window can be a lifesaver. Instead of the usual 16-hour fast, opt for a 10-hour fast. This way, you're still reaping some benefits of fasting without putting additional strain on your body. Incorporate stress-reduction techniques like deep breathing exercises, yoga, or even a short walk to help manage your stress levels. This balance between maintaining your fasting practice and managing stress can make the whole process feel more sustainable.

When dealing with illness, it's essential to give your body the rest and support it needs. If you're feeling under the weather, consider pausing your fasting routine to allow your body to recover. Focus on staying hydrated and consuming nutrient-rich foods that support healing. If you decide to continue fasting, shorten your fasting periods and ensure you're getting plenty of fluids and nutrients during your eating windows. This approach allows your body to focus on recovery while still maintaining some of the benefits of fasting.

8.6 LONG-TERM SUSTAINABILITY OF INTERMITTENT FASTING

You've been practicing intermittent fasting for a while now, and it's become a comfortable part of your routine. But as we all know, life has a funny way of throwing curveballs. Maybe you've taken up a new hobby that demands more energy, or perhaps you've noticed changes in your health that require a different approach. This is where evolving your fasting practice over time becomes crucial. Just as you wouldn't wear the same pair of shoes for every occasion, your fasting routine should adapt to fit your current needs and lifestyle. As you age, your nutritional and energy requirements change, and your fasting schedule should reflect that. For instance, you might find that a shorter fasting window works better for you now than it did a few years ago. The key is to stay flexible and open to making adjustments that align with your health status and personal goals.

Incorporating regular reviews of your fasting practice can help ensure it remains effective and sustainable. Think of it as a health check-up for your eating habits. Set aside time annually or biannually to assess how your fasting routine is working for you. Are you still feeling the benefits, or have you hit a plateau? Have there been any changes in your health that might require a different approach? Regular reviews allow you to make necessary adjustments based on your current situation and any new scientific findings. For example, if recent research suggests a different fasting method might be more beneficial for women over 50, you'll be in a good position to try it out. Keeping track of your progress and being willing to tweak your routine can help you maintain the benefits of intermittent fasting in the long run.

Fostering a flexible mindset is crucial for the long-term sustainability of intermittent fasting. Life is unpredictable, and sticking rigidly to a plan that no longer serves you can lead to frustration and burnout. Embrace the idea that it's okay to make changes. Maybe you need to shorten your fasting window during particularly busy or stressful times, or perhaps you decide to take a break from fasting altogether for a period. Being flexible doesn't mean you're giving up; it means you're listening to your body and doing what's best for your overall well-being. A flexible mindset allows you to adapt your fasting practices to fit your life, rather than forcing your life to fit your fasting schedule.

Creating lifelong habits that integrate intermittent fasting with other healthy behaviors can help make it a permanent part of your lifestyle. Think of intermittent fasting as one piece of a larger puzzle that includes regular physical activity, stress management, and a balanced diet. For instance, pairing your fasting routine with a consistent exercise schedule can enhance the benefits of both. Whether it's a daily walk, yoga session, or strength training, regular physical activity can help you maintain muscle mass, boost your metabolism, and improve your overall health. Similarly, incorporating stress management techniques like meditation, deep breathing exercises, or even hobbies that bring you joy can complement your fasting routine by helping you stay calm and focused.

To integrate intermittent fasting into your lifestyle permanently, start by making small, manageable changes. Gradually build up to a fasting schedule that feels sustainable and fits seamlessly into your daily life. For example, if you're new to fasting, start with a shorter fasting window and gradually increase it as you become more comfortable. The same goes for other healthy behaviors. Introduce new activities or habits one at a time, allowing yourself to adjust and find what works best for you. Over time, these small changes can add up to significant improvements in your health and well-being.

As you navigate the ups and downs of life, remember that the goal is to create a balanced, healthy lifestyle that supports your well-being. Intermittent fasting is a powerful tool, but it's not the only one. By integrating it with other healthy habits and staying flexible, you can maintain the benefits of fasting and enjoy a healthier, more vibrant life.

Next, we'll delve into the importance of community and social life in maintaining a sustainable fasting practice, and how to navigate social settings without compromising your health goals.

9

COMMUNITY AND SOCIAL LIFE

I magine this: You're at a lively dinner party, the aroma of delicious food wafting through the air, and everyone is toasting to a wonderful evening. You're halfway through your fasting window and suddenly, the host offers you a decadent slice of chocolate cake. You smile politely, your stomach growling in protest, and think, "How do I navigate this without derailing my progress?" Social settings can feel like a minefield when you're practicing intermittent fasting, but with a bit of planning and a few tricks up your sleeve, you can enjoy these gatherings without compromising your goals.

9.1 INTERMITTENT FASTING IN SOCIAL SETTINGS: TIPS AND TRICKS

One of the best strategies for handling social events while fasting is planning ahead. Before heading out, take a few minutes to check the restaurant menu online. Look for options that align with your eating window and dietary preferences. This way, you can make informed choices and avoid the pressure of last-minute decisions that might not align with your fasting goals. If the event is at someone's home, consider eating a small, nutritious meal beforehand. This can help curb your appetite and reduce the temptation to overeat when you arrive. Think of it as setting yourself up for success, much like a seasoned traveler plans their itinerary to ensure a smooth journey.

Now, let's talk about choosing fasting-friendly activities. Social gatherings don't always have to revolve around food. Suggest alternative activities that allow you to enjoy the company of friends and family without the focus being on eating. How about a scenic walk in the park, where you can chat and enjoy nature? Or perhaps attending a local workshop or visiting a museum? These activities not only provide a change of pace but also offer enriching experiences that don't involve food. Plus, you might discover new interests and hobbies along the way. It's like giving your social life a delightful makeover, one that aligns with your health goals.

Handling questions and peer pressure about not eating at social events can be tricky, but it's all about confidence and clear communication. When someone offers you food outside your eating window, a polite but firm response works wonders. You might say, "Thank you so much, but I'm not hungry right now," or "I'm following a new eating plan and I feel great about it." Most people will respect your choices if you present them confidently. And for the persistent ones, a little humor can help defuse the situation. A lighthearted, "I'm saving room for that amazing conversation we're about to have," can shift the focus away from food and onto more engaging topics.

Mindful eating in social contexts is another powerful tool. When you do eat at social gatherings, focus on the experience rather than the quantity of food. Take the time to savor each bite, enjoying the flavors, textures, and aromas. Engage in conversations and really listen to what others are saying. This not only enhances your social experience but also helps you eat more mindfully. You'll find that you enjoy your food more and feel satisfied with less. It's about making the meal a part of the experience, not the main event. Think of it as practicing the art of being present, where each moment is savored, much like a fine wine.

Social Event Checklist

1. **Check the Menu**: Look up restaurant menus in advance to find options that fit your eating window.
2. **Eat Beforehand**: Have a small, nutritious meal before the event to curb your appetite.
3. **Suggest Activities**: Propose non-food-centric activities like a walk, workshop, or museum visit.
4. **Polite Decline**: Have a polite but firm response ready for food offers.
5. **Mindful Eating**: Focus on savoring each bite and enjoying the company around you.

Navigating social events while intermittent fasting doesn't have to be a daunting task. With these tips, you can maintain your fasting routine while still enjoying the social interactions that make life rich and fulfilling. Remember, it's all about balance and making choices that align with your goals while also allowing you to live fully and joyfully.

9.2 COMMUNICATING YOUR FASTING LIFESTYLE TO OTHERS

Imagine this: You're at a family gathering, and your sister, who's always been a bit of a foodie, gives you a puzzled look as you pass on the appetizers. "What's this fasting thing you're doing?" she asks, clearly intrigued but a bit skeptical. This is your moment to shine! Educating friends and family about intermittent fasting can be a game-changer. Start by providing them with basic information. Explain that intermittent fasting is not about starving yourself, but about timing your meals to optimize health benefits. You might say something like, "Intermittent fasting helps me manage my weight and energy levels by giving my body a break from constant digestion. It's backed by science and has been shown to improve everything from insulin sensitivity to cognitive function." By framing it as a health choice rather than a restrictive diet, you can foster understanding and support.

Setting clear boundaries with loved ones is crucial to maintaining your focus and commitment to fasting. Picture this: You've just started your fasting window, and suddenly, your partner suggests a late-night snack while watching your favorite show. It's tempting, right? Here's where setting boundaries comes in. You can gently explain to your partner that you've committed to a fasting schedule and that it's important for your health. A simple, "I've started my fasting window, but I'd love to join you with a cup of herbal tea instead," can go a long way. Clear boundaries help you stay on track and communicate your needs without causing friction. It's about creating an environment where your health goals are respected and supported.

Now, let's tackle the elephant in the room: dealing with skepticism. We all have that one friend or family member who's quick to question our choices. The trick is to respond with factual information and a dash of confidence. For example, if someone says, "Isn't fasting bad for your metabolism?" you can calmly reply, "Actually, studies have shown that intermittent fasting can improve metabolic health by enhancing insulin sensitivity and promoting fat loss." Addressing common misconceptions with solid facts not only educates, but also shows that you've done your homework. And if they're still skeptical? That's okay. You're not here to convince everyone, just to share what's working for you.

Sharing personal benefits is another powerful way to make intermittent fasting relatable and accepted. Think back to the improvements you've noticed since you started fasting. Maybe you've lost a few pounds, your energy levels are more stable, or your mood has improved. Share these positive changes with your loved ones. You might say, "Since I started intermittent fasting, I've felt more energetic and less bloated. It's really made a difference in my daily life." Personal stories are incredibly compelling because they add a human element to the conversation. They show that intermittent fasting isn't just a theoretical concept but a practical, beneficial lifestyle change.

For those particularly interested in the science, you can mention the research backing intermittent fasting. Studies from reputable sources such as Johns Hopkins Medicine highlight benefits like improved heart health, better memory, and even potential protection against diseases like type 2 diabetes. Sharing these insights can help skeptical friends and family understand that intermittent fasting is not just another fad but a well-researched approach to health.

Communicating your fasting lifestyle doesn't have to be a daunting task. It's about educating, setting clear boundaries, addressing skepticism with facts, and sharing your personal experiences. By approaching these conversations with confidence and openness, you can foster a supportive environment that respects your health choices.

9.3 BALANCING FASTING AND FAMILY OBLIGATIONS

Finding harmony between intermittent fasting and family life can feel a bit like juggling flaming torches while riding a unicycle. But don't worry, it's entirely doable with a bit of planning and a sprinkle of creativity. One of the simplest ways to incorporate family meals into your fasting schedule is by aligning your eating window with family dinner times. For instance, if your family typically eats dinner at 6 PM, you might set your eating window from 2 PM to 8 PM. This way, you can enjoy dinner with everyone and still stick to your fasting plan. It's a win-win. You get to participate fully in the family meal without feeling like you're missing out or making things awkward.

Creating fasting-compatible family meals doesn't have to be a Herculean task. Think about dishes that are easily adjustable to fit both fasting and non-fasting members of the family. For example, a big salad bar allows everyone to customize their plates. You can load yours with greens, lean proteins, and healthy fats, while the kids might opt for some extra croutons or cheese. Another idea is to prepare a main dish like grilled chicken or fish, and then offer a variety of sides such as roasted vegetables, quinoa, or rice. This ensures that everyone gets what they need without requiring you to make separate meals. It's like being a culinary chameleon, adapting seamlessly to everyone's tastes and dietary requirements.

Educating family members about intermittent fasting can foster a supportive environment and reduce any potential friction. Start by explaining the health benefits in simple terms. You might say, "Intermittent fasting helps me manage my weight and energy levels, and it's backed by science." For children, you can liken it to the way superheroes need to recharge their powers. "Just like Spiderman needs to take a break to regain his strength, Mom needs her fasting window to stay healthy and strong." This approach not only informs, but also engages them in a way they can understand and respect. It's about creating allies rather than critics in your household.

Handling differing dietary needs can be a bit of a balancing act, but with a little ingenuity, it's entirely manageable. Consider the varying dietary preferences and needs within your household. Maybe your partner loves carbs, while you're focusing on lean proteins and veggies. Preparing versatile dishes that can be tweaked easily is key. Think of a taco night where everyone can build their own tacos. You can opt for a lettuce wrap filled with grilled chicken and avocado, while others might go for traditional shells and toppings. This way, everyone feels included, and you maintain your fasting goals without feeling like a short-order cook.

Imagine a Sunday brunch where the family gathers around the table, and instead of the usual carb-laden options, you've prepared a spread that caters to everyone. There are scrambled eggs, avocado toast on whole grain bread, fresh fruit, and yogurt parfaits. You can enjoy a hearty meal that fits within your eating window, while the kids and your partner can indulge in their favorites. This approach not only keeps you on track but also shows your family that healthy eating can be delicious and satisfying for everyone. It's about finding that sweet spot where your fasting lifestyle and family needs intersect smoothly.

When it comes to managing a household with differing dietary needs, communication is your best friend. Have open discussions about everyone's preferences and find common ground. Maybe your partner loves pasta, but you're avoiding carbs. You can prepare a pasta dish with a side of zoodles (zucchini noodles) for yourself. This way, everyone gets to enjoy their meal without feeling deprived or left out. It's about finding creative solutions that honor each person's dietary choices.

Balancing fasting and family obligations requires a bit of finesse, but it's entirely possible. With thoughtful planning, creative meal preparation, and open communication, you can maintain your fasting lifestyle while ensuring that family meals remain a time of connection and joy. It's about creating a harmonious environment where everyone feels supported and nourished, both physically and emotionally.

9.4 BUILDING A SUPPORT NETWORK OF FELLOW FASTERS

Imagine this: You're sitting at home, sipping on your favorite herbal tea, and scrolling through social media. Suddenly, you stumble upon a group dedicated to intermittent fasting, full of women sharing their experiences, tips, and encouragement. You think, "This is exactly what I need!" Finding local and online fasting communities can be a game-changer. Start by searching for forums, Facebook groups, or local meetups where you can connect with others on the same path. These communities are treasure troves of shared wisdom and support. They offer a space where you can ask questions, share your victories, and even vent about the challenges. It's like having a group of friends who just get it, making the whole process feel less isolating and more communal.

The benefits of having a support network are numerous. Firstly, it's incredibly motivating to see others succeeding and overcoming the same hurdles you face. It can inspire you to keep going, even when the going gets tough. Shared wisdom is another gem — members often share tips and strategies that you might not have thought of, like new recipes or ways to curb cravings. And let's not forget the feeling of being understood. Sometimes, just knowing that someone else has experienced the same struggles can be a huge relief. This sense of camaraderie can significantly enhance your adherence to your fasting routine. It's like having a cheerleading squad that's always rooting for your success.

Participating in group fasting challenges can add a fun and competitive element to your routine. These challenges often involve setting collective goals, like completing a 24-hour fast once a week or sticking to a particular fasting window for a month. The element of competition can make fasting more engaging and exciting. Plus, knowing that others are right there with you, facing the same challenges, can boost your commitment. It's like joining a workout class where everyone's energy and determination fuel your own. The shared experience of pushing through a challenge can create a strong bond among participants, making fasting feel less like a solitary endeavor and more like a team sport.

Creating your own support group is another fantastic option if you can't find one that suits your needs. Start by reaching out to friends, family, or colleagues who might be interested in intermittent fasting. You'd be surprised how many people are curious about it but haven't taken the plunge because they lack support. Once you have a few interested individuals, set up regular meetings—these could be in-person or virtual, depending on everyone's preference. Structure the meetings to include sharing experiences, discussing new research, and setting collective goals. You might even want to invite guest speakers, like nutritionists or experienced fasters, to provide additional insights. Having a structured yet flexible agenda can keep the meetings productive and engaging.

When setting up your support group, consider incorporating elements that make participation enjoyable and rewarding. For example, you could start each meeting with a round of "win of the week," where everyone shares a positive experience or achievement related to fasting. This not only starts the meeting on a positive note but also highlights the progress being made. You could also organize mini-challenges within the group, like who can come up with the most creative fasting-friendly recipe. These activities can make the meetings something to look forward to, rather than just another commitment on the calendar.

Building a support network, whether through existing communities or by creating your own, can make a significant difference in your intermittent fasting journey. It provides a sense of belonging, offers valuable resources, and turns what could be a solitary practice into a shared adventure. Knowing you have a group of people who understand and support you can make all the difference in staying committed to your health goals. It's about creating a community that lifts you up, celebrates your victories, and helps you navigate the challenges with confidence and joy.

9.5 CELEBRATING FESTIVITIES WITHOUT BREAKING YOUR FAST

Holidays and special occasions often revolve around food, making it tricky to stick to your fasting schedule. However, with a bit of foresight, you can navigate these events without feeling deprived. One effective strategy is to choose which events to align with your eating windows. If you know you'll be attending a holiday dinner that starts at 6 PM, adjust your fasting schedule so that your eating window includes that time. This way, you can fully participate in the meal without breaking your fast. It's like creating a custom plan that fits both your social life and your health goals. Planning special meals that fit within your fasting schedule can also help. You might prepare a nutritious, satisfying dish that you can bring to the event, ensuring there's something you can eat that aligns with your fasting plan. This not only keeps you on track but also adds to the festive table.

Celebrations don't always have to center around food. Alternative celebration ideas can be just as enjoyable and perhaps even more memorable. Consider organizing games, outings, or gift exchanges that everyone can enjoy, regardless of their eating schedules. For instance, you might plan a fun game night with family and friends, complete with board games and laughter, instead of a heavy meal. Or how about a holiday outing, like a walk through a beautifully lit park or a visit to a local museum? These activities shift the focus from food to shared experiences and create lasting memories without the calorie overload. It's a refreshing way to celebrate that keeps everyone engaged and active.

Adjusting fasting schedules temporarily to accommodate special occasions is another practical approach. Don't be afraid to tweak your fasting window for a day to fit a special event. If you usually fast from 8 PM to noon the next day but have a late-night celebration, consider starting your fast later and ending it later the next day. This flexibility allows you to enjoy the occasion without feeling restricted. The key is to return to your regular schedule afterward. Think of it as taking a small detour on your fasting path, knowing you'll get back on track soon. It's about maintaining a balance between your fasting discipline and life's celebratory moments.

During festive periods, adopting a flexible and forgiving mindset is crucial. It's easy to get caught up in the strictness of fasting, but remember that these celebrations are about joy and togetherness. Allow yourself to enjoy the moment and be present with your loved ones. If you indulge a bit more than planned, don't stress about it. Life is meant to be enjoyed, and one day of deviation won't derail your progress. Emphasize the importance of balance and self-compassion. After all, the goal is to create a sustainable lifestyle that enhances your well-being without feeling like a burden. Think of it as giving yourself permission to enjoy life's special moments while keeping an eye on your long-term health goals.

As we wrap up this chapter, it's clear that community and social life play a significant role in maintaining a sustainable fasting routine. By planning ahead, communicating your lifestyle, balancing family obligations, building a support network, and navigating festive periods with flexibility, you can enjoy a fulfilling social life without compromising your health goals. Remember, intermittent fasting is not just a diet; it's a lifestyle choice that can harmonize with your daily activities and special occasions alike.

Next, we'll explore how to continue your fasting journey, evolving your strategy as you age, staying informed about new research, and inspiring others by sharing your story.

10

CONTINUING YOUR FASTING JOURNEY

Picture this: You're sitting in your favorite armchair, sipping on a cup of herbal tea, and reflecting on how far you've come with intermittent fasting. You remember the initial jitters, the hunger pangs, and the skepticism. Now, you're here, feeling more in tune with your body and your health than ever before. But the journey doesn't stop here. As we age, our bodies continue to change, and it's important to evolve our fasting strategies to keep up with these changes.

10.1 EVOLVING YOUR FASTING STRATEGY AS YOU AGE

Aging is like navigating a winding road with unexpected turns. One day, you're cruising along, and the next, you hit a bump that throws you off balance. Understanding how aging affects our metabolism, hormone levels, and energy needs can help us adjust our intermittent fasting practices to stay on track. As we age, our metabolism tends to slow down. This isn't just about burning fewer calories; it's about how our body processes and uses energy. Hormonal changes, such as decreased levels of estrogen and progesterone in women, also play a significant role. These shifts can affect everything from our weight to our mood and energy levels.

Intermittent fasting can help mitigate some of these changes, but it's important to adapt the duration and type of fasting as we age. For example, the 16/8 method, where you fast for 16 hours and eat within an 8-hour window, might have been a breeze in your 40s. However, in your 50s and beyond, you might find that a shorter fasting window, like 14/10, is more manageable and still provides benefits. The key is to listen to your body and adjust accordingly. If you find that longer fasts leave you feeling drained or irritable, it's okay to shorten the fasting period. Flexibility is your friend here.

Incorporating preventive health measures is another crucial aspect of evolving your fasting strategy. Regular health screenings can help you monitor your blood pressure, cholesterol levels, and other vital health markers. These screenings provide valuable insights into how your body is responding to intermittent fasting and whether any adjustments are needed. Additionally, dietary adjustments can play a significant role in addressing age-related health concerns. For example, increasing your intake of calcium and vitamin D can help maintain bone health, which is particularly important as we age. Including more fiber in your diet can aid digestion and support heart health.

Let's look at a couple of case studies to illustrate how adapting fasting strategies can lead to long-term success. Meet Karen, a 55-year-old teacher who started intermittent fasting to manage her weight and energy levels. Initially, Karen followed the 16/8 method but found that it left her feeling fatigued by midday. After consulting with her healthcare provider, she switched to the 14/10 method and incorporated more protein and healthy fats into her meals. This adjustment not only improved her energy levels but also helped her maintain a steady weight.

Then there's Linda, a 62-year-old retiree who struggled with high blood pressure and cholesterol. Linda started with the 5:2 method, where she restricted her calorie intake to 500-600 calories on two non-consecutive days each week. However, she found it challenging to stick to such a low-calorie count. After some trial and error, she switched to a modified version of the 5:2 method, where she consumed 800 calories on fasting days. This slight increase made the fasting days more manageable and still provided significant health benefits. Over time, Linda's blood pressure and cholesterol levels improved, and she felt more in control of her health.

These examples highlight the importance of tailoring your fasting strategy to fit your unique needs and circumstances. What worked for you in the past might need tweaking as you age, and that's perfectly okay. The goal is to find a sustainable and effective approach that supports your overall well-being.

Understanding the role of hormone levels in intermittent fasting is also critical. Hormones like estrogen and progesterone decline with age, which can impact everything from your metabolism to your mood. Incorporating hormone-supportive foods into your diet can help mitigate some of these effects. Foods rich in phytoestrogens, such as flaxseeds, soy products, and legumes, can help balance hormone levels. Additionally, healthy fats like those found in avocados, nuts, and olive oil, as well as Omega-3 fatty acids from sources like salmon and mackerel, can support overall hormonal health.

Regular exercise is another preventive measure that can complement intermittent fasting. Engaging in both aerobic and resistance exercises can improve insulin sensitivity, boost metabolism, and support muscle mass maintenance. As we age, maintaining muscle mass becomes increasingly important for overall health and mobility. Weight training and bodyweight exercises are excellent ways to achieve this. Even simple activities like walking or swimming can make a significant difference.

Let's not forget the importance of staying hydrated. As we age, our sense of thirst may diminish, making it easy to become dehydrated without realizing it. Drinking enough water is crucial for overall health and can help prevent common issues like constipation and urinary tract infections. Herbal teas and infused water can make staying hydrated more enjoyable.

One of the most empowering aspects of intermittent fasting is that it's a flexible tool. You can adjust your fasting schedule, meal composition, and exercise routine to fit your evolving needs. This adaptability makes it a sustainable practice that can support you throughout different stages of life.

As you continue your fasting journey, remember that it's not about perfection but about progress. Celebrate your successes, no matter how small, and be kind to yourself on days when things don't go as planned. The goal is to create a lifestyle that enhances your well-being and brings you joy. Intermittent fasting is just one piece of the puzzle, and when combined with other healthy habits, it can lead to a more vibrant and fulfilling life.

10.2 STAYING INFORMED: CONTINUAL LEARNING AND ADAPTATION

Picture this: You're sipping your morning coffee, scrolling through the latest health news, when you stumble upon a headline about new research on intermittent fasting. You're intrigued, but also a bit overwhelmed. How do you keep up with all this information? Staying informed about the latest research is crucial for adapting your fasting practices to ensure they remain effective and safe.

To stay updated, start with trustworthy sources. Websites like the National Institutes of Health (NIH) and academic journals such as "The Journal of Clinical Endocrinology & Metabolism" are gold mines of reliable information. Subscribing to health newsletters from reputable organizations can also keep you in the loop. Podcasts and webinars featuring experts in nutrition and gerontology are another great way to absorb new information. These resources often break down complex studies into digestible, actionable insights.

In addition to these resources, consider joining online forums or social media groups dedicated to intermittent fasting. These communities can offer valuable tips, share the latest research, and provide support. Engaging in discussions with like-minded individuals can spark new ideas and help you stay motivated. Remember, the more you know, the better equipped you are to make informed decisions about your health.

Personal health tracking tools are another excellent way to gather and interpret data about your fasting journey. Apps like MyFitnessPal and LifeSum can help you track your food intake, fasting windows, and even your exercise routines. These apps often come with features that allow you to log how you're feeling physically and emotionally, providing a holistic view of your health. By consistently logging this data, you can start to see patterns and identify what works best for you. Did you notice that you feel more energetic when you break your fast with a protein-rich meal? Or perhaps you sleep better when your last meal of the day includes complex carbohydrates? These insights can help you fine-tune your fasting practices for optimal results.

Understanding how to interpret this data is key. Look for trends rather than isolated incidents. If you felt sluggish on a particular day, consider what you ate, how you slept, and your stress levels. Cross-reference this with your fasting schedule to see if there's a connection. Over time, you'll develop a clearer picture of how different variables affect your health. This personalized approach ensures that your fasting practices are tailored to your unique needs and circumstances.

Adapting to new knowledge is an ongoing process. As new research emerges, be open to making adjustments to your fasting routine. For example, if a new study suggests that shorter fasting windows are particularly beneficial for post-menopausal women, consider experimenting with a 14/10 schedule instead of your usual 16/8. Keep a journal to document how these changes affect you. This trial-and-error approach allows you to find what works best for your body.

Engaging with professional guidance is another crucial aspect of continual learning and adaptation. Regular consultations with healthcare providers can help you tailor your fasting strategy based on your health status and any new medical advice. For instance, if you're diagnosed with a new health condition or start a new medication, your healthcare provider can offer personalized recommendations to ensure your fasting practices remain safe and effective. They can also provide insights into any new research that might be particularly relevant to you.

Don't hesitate to seek out specialists who can offer more targeted advice. Nutritionists, endocrinologists, and gerontologists can provide valuable insights into how intermittent fasting interacts with your specific health needs. Building a relationship with these professionals ensures you have a reliable source of information and support as you navigate your fasting journey.

Remember, the world of health and nutrition is constantly evolving. What we know today may change tomorrow, and that's okay. The goal is to stay adaptable and open to new information. By keeping up with the latest research, using personal health tracking tools, and engaging with professional guidance, you can ensure your fasting practices continue to support your health and well-being.

To make this process more interactive, consider setting aside a little time each week to review new studies or articles. Make it a routine—perhaps a Sunday morning ritual with a cup of tea. This not only keeps you informed but also reinforces your commitment to your health.

Incorporating new knowledge doesn't mean overhauling your entire routine every time a new study comes out. Small, incremental changes are often more sustainable and effective. For instance, if you learn that a particular nutrient can enhance the benefits of fasting, start by incorporating foods rich in that nutrient into your meals. Monitor how you feel and adjust as necessary.

10.3 INSPIRING OTHERS BY SHARING YOUR FASTING JOURNEY

Imagine you're sitting at a coffee shop with a friend, and she can't help but notice how much more energetic and vibrant you seem. She asks, "What's your secret?" This is your moment to share your intermittent fasting story. By opening up about your personal experiences, you can inspire others to explore fasting for themselves. Sharing your journey doesn't have to be a grand gesture; it can be as simple as a heartfelt conversation or a casual social media post. Talk about the challenges you faced, the strategies that worked, and the victories you celebrated. Your story is unique and powerful, and it can motivate others to take that first step towards better health.

When it comes to educational outreach, the key is to be informative without being intrusive. Think about how you felt when you first learned about intermittent fasting. You probably had a lot of questions and maybe even some doubts. Approach others with empathy, understanding that they might be in the same boat. Start by sharing evidence-based benefits, such as improved energy levels, better mood, and sustainable weight loss. Use simple, relatable language and avoid jargon that might overwhelm or confuse. Personal anecdotes can be incredibly effective here. For example, if intermittent fasting helped you manage menopausal symptoms, share that experience. It makes the information more relatable and shows that the benefits are achievable.

Creating engaging content can amplify your reach and inspire a larger community. If you enjoy writing, consider starting a blog where you document your fasting experiences, share tips, and provide recipes. Social media platforms like Instagram or Facebook are also great for sharing daily updates, meal ideas, and motivational quotes. You don't have to be a professional writer or photographer to create content that resonates. Authenticity is your best asset. Share real-life moments, both the triumphs and the setbacks. This honesty fosters a sense of community and support among your followers. If speaking is more your style, consider giving presentations at local community centers or health clubs. You could even host webinars or live Q&A sessions online to reach a broader audience.

Mentoring and participating in support groups can be incredibly rewarding. Think back to when you started your fasting journey —having someone to guide you through the ups and downs would have been invaluable, right? By becoming a mentor, you can offer that support to others. Share your knowledge, provide encouragement, and celebrate their successes. Support groups, whether in-person or online, provide a platform for people to share their experiences, ask questions, and find motivation. Leading a support group can be as simple as organizing weekly meetups where members discuss their progress and challenges. You can also create a private Facebook group or WhatsApp chat where members can stay connected and support each other daily. Mentoring and support groups are powerful tools for personal growth and community building. They help you stay accountable while inspiring others to achieve their health goals.

Imagine the ripple effect of your influence. By sharing your fasting journey, educating others, creating engaging content, and participating in support groups, you're not just improving your own health; you're empowering a community. Each person you inspire can, in turn, inspire others, creating a network of individuals committed to better health and well-being.

As you continue to inspire others, remember that everyone's journey is unique. What works for one person might not work for another, and that's okay. Encourage others to experiment, listen to their bodies, and find what works best for them. Remind them that intermittent fasting is not a one-size-fits-all solution but a flexible tool that can be tailored to fit their individual needs and lifestyles. By fostering a supportive and inclusive community, you can help others discover the transformative power of intermittent fasting.

Sharing your story, educating others, creating content, and mentoring are not just ways to inspire others—they're also ways to deepen your own commitment to intermittent fasting. As you share your knowledge and experiences, you'll find that you become more mindful of your own practices. You'll stay motivated and engaged, knowing that you're making a positive impact on the lives of others. This mutual support and inspiration create a cycle of growth and improvement that benefits everyone involved.

In summary, your personal fasting journey has the potential to inspire and empower others. By sharing your story, educating your community, creating engaging content, and participating in or leading support groups, you can make a meaningful difference in the lives of those around you. This chapter has explored the various ways you can share your journey and the impact it can have. As you continue to evolve your fasting practices and stay informed, remember that your experiences and knowledge are valuable resources that can inspire and support others on their path to better health.

SPREAD THE WORD

Congratulations on completing this book and honing all the knowledge you need to make intermittent fasting a safe, pleasurable, and flavor-filled journey toward better health. I can imagine you're excited about trying out new workouts and recipes and building a support network of fellow fasters. Before you go, however, please leave a quick review of this book if you haven't done so already. This alone will help grow the community of women over 50 who are keen to feel strong, energetic, and vibrant.

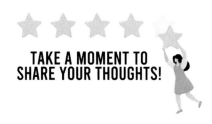

TAKE A MOMENT TO SHARE YOUR THOUGHTS!

Thanks for your help. May you thrive on the path to optimal health and inspire many others to share your fasting journey!

Scan the QR code below

CONCLUSION

Well, here we are at the end of our journey together, but don't worry—it's just the beginning of a new chapter in your life. Remember when we started this book? We set out to explore intermittent fasting not as a fleeting diet trend but as a sustainable, holistic approach to improving health, managing menopausal symptoms, and enhancing your quality of life. And gosh, haven't we covered some ground?

We've delved into how intermittent fasting can transform your life, especially as a woman over 50. From boosting your energy levels and elevating your mood to managing stress and improving sleep quality—this isn't just about shedding a few pounds. It's about reclaiming control over your health and well-being during a phase of life that often feels like a rollercoaster.

One thing we've emphasized throughout is our commitment to science-backed research. We didn't just throw around fancy terms and theories; we grounded our advice in solid evidence. We talked about how intermittent fasting impacts your metabolism, enhances autophagy (that's the cell-cleaning process), and helps balance your hormones. All these nerdy-sounding concepts have real, tangible benefits tailored just for you.

But let's not forget the practical side of things. We've shared customizable fasting schedules so you can find what fits your lifestyle best. We've talked about nutritional strategies, like incorporating nutrient-dense foods and anti-inflammatory ingredients, to support your fasting journey. We even tackled exercise recommendations, so you're not left wondering what kind of physical activity pairs well with fasting. And yes, we discussed how to navigate social situations and emotional challenges without feeling like you're missing out on life's pleasures.

The beauty of intermittent fasting is that it's not one-size-fits-all. The guidance in this book is meant to be personalized. Your health profile, your lifestyle, your preferences—they all matter. So, feel empowered to adapt the information to suit your unique situation. It's your journey, and you're in the driver's seat.

We've also highlighted that intermittent fasting's benefits go far beyond weight loss. It's about feeling more vibrant, more energetic, and more in control of your health. From improving cardiovascular health to potentially delaying the aging process and preventing chronic diseases, the holistic health benefits are immense.

But here's the thing: The science of fasting is always evolving. New research is coming out all the time. So, stay curious and keep learning. Be open to adjusting your fasting practices as you age or as new scientific insights emerge. This journey is ongoing, and staying informed will only help you make better decisions for your health.

And don't keep this transformative experience to yourself! Share your journey with others. Whether it's through social media, community groups, or just chatting with friends, your story can inspire others to consider intermittent fasting. You might be the spark that encourages someone else to take control of their health.

Now, here's my call to action: Take the first step on your intermittent fasting journey. Approach it with patience and flexibility. Remember, this isn't about perfection; it's about progress and making positive changes for your health and well-being. Embrace the process, celebrate the small victories, and be kind to yourself on the tough days.

Acknowledge that this journey is personal and evolving. There will be challenges—heck, there might be days when you want to throw in the towel. But see these challenges as opportunities for growth and learning. Every step, every stumble, is part of your story.

I want to express my deepest gratitude to you for embarking on this journey with me. Your commitment to exploring intermittent fasting and improving your health is truly inspiring. Remember, the path to better health is rewarding, filled with discovery, empowerment, and a whole lot of personal victories.

You've got this. Here's to a healthier, happier you! Cheers!

30 DELICIOUS INTERMITTENT FASTING MEAL IDEAS

TACO SALAD RECIPE

Ingredients:

- Two cans of kidney beans (drained)
- One head of iceberg lettuce (chopped)
- One can of black olives (sliced)
- Two or three tomatoes, depending on the size (chopped)
- 1 cup of mayonnaise
- 1 cup of ketchup
- 1 packet of taco seasoning
- 2 bags of Fritos chips (or equivalent)
- Optional ingredients
  - Avocado, sliced
  - Burger, pan-fried in oil with chopped onions.

Instructions:

1. Prepare ingredients: Drain liquid from kidney beans; wash and chop lettuce; drain liquid from black olives and chop them; wash and chop tomatoes; etc.
2. Add the kidney beans, lettuce, black olives and tomatoes to a large bowl, and mix. (Add optional ingredients as desired.)
3. Add the mayonnaise, ketchup, and packet of taco seasoning to the bowl, and stir thoroughly.

4. Add the Fritos immediately before serving. If you add them too early, they will get soggy quickly. Stir the Fritos in so that they are coated with the dressing mixture.

PEA SOUP RECIPE

Ingredients:

- 1 pound bag of dry green split peas, rinsed
- 2 quarts of water
- 2 stalks of celery, chopped
- 2 large carrots, peeled and chopped
- 1 large onion, peeled and chopped
- ½ teaspoon marjoram
- ½ teaspoon thyme
- 1 teaspoon salt

Instructions:

1. Pour the bag of dry green split peas into a large pot, and rinse thoroughly, making sure to remove any rocks or debris.
2. Add 2 quarts of water to the pot of green split peas, and put on the stove, bringing it to a boil.
3. As the peas come to a boil, rinse and chop celery. Rinse, peel, and chop the carrots and onion. Add the vegetables to the pot. Stir.
4. Add marjoram, thyme, and salt to the pot. Stir.
5. After all the ingredients come to a boil, reduce to a simmer. Cook for about 45 to 60 minutes, or until the peas and vegetables are tender. Stir periodically.
6. Add the soup mixture into a blender, and blend on high until thoroughly pureed. Serve and enjoy!

KALE SALAD RECIPE

Ingredients:

- Two large bunches of kale
- ½ cup of Pure maple syrup* (note: it must be pure maple syrup, not fake artificial syrup)
- ½ cup of olive oil*
- ½ tablespoon to 1 tablespoon of sesame oil

Instructions:

1. Wash the kale thoroughly.
2. Remove the stems and break the leaves into bite-size chunks. Place into a large salad bowl.
3. In a small bowl, mix the olive oil, maple syrup, and sesame oil very thoroughly. Oil and maple syrup don't like to mix easily, so really mix it well.
4. Pour the dressing mixture over the kale, and then use clean hands to massage in the dressing. Massaging the dressing into the leaves helps to reduce the toughness of the kale, as well as infuse the dressing into the leaves.
5. Add toppings of your choice. Ideas include but are not limited to:
   a. Very thinly sliced apples (preferably Pink Lady apples for tartness)
   b. Toasted slivered almonds or other nuts
   c. Thinly sliced red (purple) onions (make sure they're not too spicy or it will affect the overall taste of the salad)
   d. Dried cranberries

- If you have a lot of kale and need to make more dressing, just make sure that it's equal parts olive oil and maple syrup.

SWEET POTATO CASSEROLE RECIPE

Ingredients:

- 1½ cups sweet potatoes [this is approximately three medium sweet potatoes]
- ½ cup sugar
- ¼ cup butter or vegan butter substitute
- 1 egg, slightly beaten (or equivalent)
- ½ cup shredded coconut
- 1/3 cup heavy cream or evaporated milk
- ½ teaspoon vanilla extract

Topping:

- ½ cup brown sugar
- ½ cup chopped pecans
- ¼ cup all-purpose flour
- ¼ cup butter or vegan butter substitute, melted
- Dash of salt

Instructions:

1. Peel and then boil sweet potatoes until soft. Drain water and mash sweet potatoes.
2. Combine mashed sweet potatoes, sugar, butter, egg, coconut, heavy cream and vanilla; mix well. Pour into buttered casserole dish. For the topping, mix brown

sugar, pecans, flour, melted butter and salt. Pour over top of sweet potato mixture.
3. Bake at 350 degrees Fahrenheit for 20 to 30 minutes. Serves approximately ten people.

EASY INDIAN DAL RECIPE

Ingredients:

- 1 large onion, diced
- Olive oil or regular oil
- 4 teaspoons curry powder
- 4 teaspoons ground cumin
- 4 teaspoons garam masala
- 4 teaspoons garlic powder (or you can use fresh garlic if you prefer)
- 1 tablespoon turmeric
- 1 to 2 teaspoons chili powder
- 2 teaspoons ground ginger (or you can use fresh ginger if you prefer)
- 2 cups of red lentils, rinsed
- Water
- 2 teaspoons salt

Instructions:

1. Dice a large onion, and sauté it in olive oil (or regular oil) until the onions are translucent. Reduce to low heat.
2. Add curry powder, cumin, garam masala, garlic powder, turmeric, chili powder, and ground ginger to the onion/oil mixture. You might have to add some more oil to saturate the spices. Make sure to stir frequently to prevent burning on the bottom of the pot. Sauté

mixture for about 3 minutes, until spices are very fragrant.

3. Add a cup of water to the pot to prevent burning.
4. Next, rinse the red lentils thoroughly to remove any small rocks or debris.
5. Add the red lentils to the pot. Add about 4 to 5 cups water. Bring to a boil.
6. After lentils have come to a boil, reduce heat and simmer on low/medium for 45 minutes. You will have to add more water from time to time, depending on how much the lentils swell. The end consistency of the dal should be like porridge - not too runny, so add water accordingly.
7. Add salt, and simmer for another 5 minutes or so to infuse the salt into the lentils.
8. Serve over rice, with Indian flatbread if you have some. Garlic naan, and malabari paratha which are all delicious with this dal
9. You can also garnish your individual serving of dal with fresh cilantro, fresh diced tomatoes, or Italian parsley etc.

VEGETARIAN FAJITAS RECIPE

Fajita Seasoning Mix Ingredients:

- 2 teaspoons chili powder
- 1 teaspoon salt
- 1 teaspoon paprika
- 1 teaspoon sugar –
- ½ teaspoon onion powder
- ½ teaspoon garlic powder
- ¼ teaspoon cayenne pepper
- ½ teaspoon ground cumin
- Optional: 1 tablespoon cornstarch

Other Fajita Ingredients:

- 1 large onion (white or yellow)
- 1 green bell pepper
- Approximately 8 ounces of fresh mushrooms
- 1 to 2 zucchinis (depending on the size)
- Approximately 10 – 12 ounces of a meat or substitute of your choice

Instructions:

1. Mix all seasoning ingredients together in a small bowl and set aside.
2. Chop up vegetables and meat substitute of your choice.
3. Sauté chopped vegetables and meat substitute in oil in a large frying pan.
4. After the veggies and meat have been sautéing for a few minutes, add the fajita seasoning mix. You may need to add some water to mix in the seasonings. If the mushrooms have been "weeping" a lot, you might not need that much water. Also, depending on the amount of your chopped vegetables, you may not need the entire mixture of fajita seasoning. Add the seasoning to taste.
5. Serve in a flour tortilla. When you're ready to use them, simply heat them in a hot skillet on the stovetop for approximately 30 seconds per side. There's nothing like a hot, freshly cooked tortilla!
6. You can add your favorite salsa and/or guacamole to your fajita wrap. But this fajita recipe is flavorful enough without the salsa and guacamole. It's up to you! Enjoy!

THE FLUFFIEST PANCAKES RECIPE

Ingredients:

- 1 cup flour
- 2 tablespoons sugar [Florida Crystals Organic Raw Cane Sugar]
- 1 tablespoon baking powder
- ½ teaspoon salt
- 1 cup soy milk [Milk of your Choice]
- 1 tablespoon lemon juice
- 1 teaspoon vanilla

Instructions:

1. In a medium bowl, add the flour, sugar, baking powder, and salt. Stir to combine.
2. In a medium bowl, add the soy milk, lemon juice, and vanilla. Stir to combine.
3. Pour the liquid mixture into the dry mixture and whisk until smooth.
4. Let batter rest for 5 minutes.
5. Pour about ½ cup of batter onto a nonstick pan or griddle over medium heat. (use spray oil on the griddle to prevent sticking.) If desired, add ingredients of your choice (i.e. pecan pieces, blueberries, white chocolate chips, regular chocolate chips, crushed pineapple and coconut flakes, etc.).
6. When the top begins to bubble, flip the pancake and cook until golden.
7. Serve warm with genuine maple syrup, berry compote, organic powdered sugar, peanut butter and apple sauce, or your favorite topping!

EASY CHIA PUDDING RECIPE

Ingredients:

- ½ cup chia seeds
- 1 ½ cups coconut milk (or a 13 ounce can of any milk is fine)
- 1 teaspoon vanilla extract
- 1 to 2 tablespoons maple syrup [if you are using unsweetened coconut milk, then you might want to add more maple syrup for sweetener.]

Instructions:

1. Add the chia seeds to a bowl. Then add the coconut milk, vanilla extract, and maple syrup. Stir thoroughly. Cover bowl and place in the refrigerator. After about a half hour or so, stir up the mixture. The chia seeds tend to float to the bottom of the bowl at the beginning; so as the mixture starts to thicken, you should stir it once or twice so that the chia seeds are more evenly dispersed throughout the pudding. Refrigerate overnight (or at least 8 hours for safety). Serve chilled, and top with a fruit of your choice. You can use fresh mango and it's a delicious combo! Fresh peaches or strawberries or other fresh fruit would also be good.

SURPRISE MUFFINS RECIPE

Ingredients:

- 1 egg (or equivalent)
- ½ cup milk or soy milk

- ¼ cup oil
- 1½ cups all-purpose flour
- ½ cup sugar [organic raw cane sugar - Florida Crystals]
- 2 teaspoons baking powder
- ½ teaspoon salt

Instructions:

1. Heat oven to 400 degrees Fahrenheit. Grease bottoms of 12 muffin cups in a muffin pan or use paper liners.
2. In a bowl, beat egg. Stir in soy milk and oil. Mix in remaining ingredients just until flour is moistened (the batter should be lumpy). Fill muffin cups half full. To each muffin cup, add 1 teaspoon of your favorite jam or jelly. Add more batter to fill the cups 2/3s full.
3. Bake 20 to 25 minutes, or until golden brown. Remove immediately from pan.
   - Yield: 1 dozen surprise muffins.
4. Tip: to truly make them surprise muffins, I use different types of jam (i.e. 4 muffins with raspberry jam, 4 with strawberry jam, and 4 with peach jam), so people don't know what type they're getting until they bite into the muffin
5. Note: You can also use this muffin batter recipe to make banana walnut muffins. Add approximately ¾ cups of chopped walnuts and approximately 1½ cups of mashed bananas to the batter and mix thoroughly. (Bananas thawed from frozen and then mashed tend to work better than fresh mashed bananas). Then spoon the batter into the muffin cups.

EASY BAKE ENERGY BITES RECIPE

Ingredients:

- 1 cup oatmeal
- ½ cup chocolate chips
- ½ cup peanut butter
- ½ cup ground flaxseed
- 1/3 cup honey
- 1 teaspoon vanilla

Instructions:

1. Mix all ingredients together thoroughly. Roll into balls (approximately 1 to 1.5 inches in diameter, a piece) and refrigerate before eating. These freeze well, if you want to save some for a snack later.

HEALTHY OAT WAFFLE RECIPE

Ingredients:

- 4 cups old-fashioned rolled oats
- 1 cup raw unsalted cashews [raw unsalted almonds works just as well!]
- ¼ cup whole wheat flour [You can substitute white flour or bread flour]
- ¼ cup oil
- 1 teaspoon salt
- 2 teaspoons vanilla [If you don't have vanilla readily available, you can substitute 1 teaspoon of maple syrup]
- 6 cups water

Instructions:

1. Place all ingredients in a blender, and blend until smooth (about 30 seconds or so).
2. The batter will be thin but will thicken. Pour into a hot, well-greased waffle iron, and cook 10 – 12 minutes until steaming stops. [For best results, spray oil on the waffle iron in between every few batches, so that the waffles don't stick to the iron.]

BLACK BEAN CHILI RECIPE

Ingredients:

- 1 medium onion
- 2 – 3 cloves of fresh garlic
- Several tablespoons of olive oil
- 1 can Vege-Burger or Redi-Burger
- 1 packet of Old El Paso Taco Seasoning Mix
- 1 can of black beans with liquid
- 1 can of Ro-Tel (ready-cut diced tomatoes w/ green chilis and spices)
- 1 can of tomato soup [you can substitute with one can of Hunt's Tomatoes Sauce]
- 1 bay leaf

Instructions:

1. Sautee onion and garlic together in olive oil in a large stockpot, until onions are translucent. Add the rest of the ingredients to the stockpot. Simmer for about 10 minutes or until done. Makes about 6 servings.

DELICIOUS CHICKEN FLORENTINE RECIPE

Ingredients:

- 4 boneless skinless chicken breasts
- Salt and freshly ground black pepper
- All-purpose flour, for dredging
- 6 tablespoons (3/4 stick) unsalted butter
- 2 tablespoons shallots, sliced
- 2 tablespoons lime juice
- 1 tablespoon chopped garlic
- 1 medium bag Fresh Spinach
- 1 1/2 cups dry white wine
- 1 cup whipping cream
- 2 branches Fresh thyme

Instructions:

1. Soak chicken in lime juice for 5 minutes then rinse with water, sprinkle the chicken with salt and pepper. Dredge the chicken in the flour to coat lightly. Shake off any excess flour. Melt 2 tablespoons of butter in a heavy large skillet over medium heat. Add the chicken and cook until brown, about 5 minutes per side. Transfer the chicken to a plate and tent with foil to keep it warm.
2. Melt 2 tablespoons of butter in the same skillet over medium heat. Add the shallots and garlic and sauté until the shallots are translucent, stirring to scrape up any browned bits on the bottom of the skillet, about 1 minute. Add the wine. Increase the heat to medium-high and boil until the liquid is reduced by half, about 3 minutes. Add the cream and boil until the sauce reduces by half, stirring often, about 3 minutes. Stir in the

parsley and fresh thyme. Season the sauce, to taste, with salt and pepper. Add the chicken and any accumulated juices to the sauce and turn the chicken to coat in the sauce.

3. Meanwhile, melt the remaining 2 tablespoons of butter in another large skillet over medium heat. Add the spinach and sauté until heated through. Season the spinach, to taste, with salt and pepper. Arrange the spinach over a platter. Place the chicken atop the spinach. Pour the sauce over and serve.

HONEY-DIJON CHICKEN MADE EASY RECIPE

Ingredients:

- 2 tablespoons honey
- 2 tablespoons Dijon mustard
- 1 tablespoon extra-virgin olive oil, plus more for grill
- 1/2 teaspoon kosher salt
- Freshly ground black pepper
- 4 boneless skinless chicken breasts, butterflied
- 1 lime, cut into wedges
- 4 tablespoon of lime Juice

Instructions:

1. Soak Chicken in lime juice for 5 minutes then rinse with warm water. In a small bowl, add the honey, mustard, 1 tablespoon of oil and salt and pepper, to taste. Mix well and put the mixture into a large plastic resealable bag. Add the chicken, seal the bag and shake to incorporate. Refrigerate at least 2 hours.
2. Preheat the grill to medium heat.

3. Remove the chicken from the bag and arrange it on a well-oiled grill. Cook until a nice crust forms on both sides, about 4 to 5 minutes per side. Let the chicken rest on a serving platter for 10 minutes before serving. Serve with lime wedges.

GRILLED CHICKEN SALAD RECIPE

Ingredients:

- 4 boneless, skinless chicken breasts
- Mixed salad greens (lettuce, spinach, arugula)
- Cherry tomatoes, halved
- 2 Limes
- Cucumber, sliced
- Red onion, thinly sliced
- Balsamic vinaigrette dressing

Instructions:

1. Preheat the grill to medium-high heat.
2. Soak chicken in lime juice for 5 minutes then rinse with warm water. Season the chicken breasts with salt and pepper.
3. Grill the chicken for about 6–8 minutes on each side or until cooked through.
4. Let the chicken rest for a few minutes, then slice it into thin strips.
5. In a large bowl, toss the mixed salad greens, cherry tomatoes, cucumber, and red onion together.
6. Drizzle the balsamic vinaigrette dressing over the salad and toss to coat.

7. Divide the salad into serving plates and top each with the grilled chicken strips. Add favorite toppings. Enjoy the deliciousness.

POST-WORKOUT OMELETTE RECIPE

Ingredients:

- 4 large eggs
- A generous handful of fresh spinach leaves
- 1/4 cup of finely diced bell peppers
- 1/4 cup of delectable, crumbled feta cheese
- Salt and pepper to tasteful perfection
- Olive oil for culinary magic
- Hint of parsley

Instructions:

1. In a bowl, beat the eggs until they attain a velvety consistency. Season them with a dash of salt and pepper, infusing them with delightful flavors.
2. Heat a drizzle of olive oil in a non-stick pan, over medium heat.
3. Add the diced bell peppers in the heated pan, sautéing them until they reach a tender state.
4. Add the fresh spinach leaves to the pan.
5. Pour the beaten eggs into the pan, skillfully spreading them.
6. Sprinkle the crumbled feta cheese upon the eggs, with the freshly diced parsley.
7. Flip the omelette over, ensuring a seamless completion.
8. Slide the omelette onto a plate and delicately fold it in half.

9. Serve warm.

TASTY AVOCADO TOAST RECIPE

Ingredients:

- 1 ripe avocado
- 2 slices of wholesome whole-grain bread
- Sliced cherry tomatoes
- A pinch of premium sea salt
- 1 Medium red Onion
- Optional garnishes: red pepper flakes, fresh parsley and a tantalizing squeeze of lemon juice

Instructions:

1. Halve the avocado, dispose of the pit, and gently scoop the velvety flesh into a bowl.
2. Employ a fork to artfully mash the avocado until it attains your preferred texture.
3. Sprinkle a pinch of the finest sea salt, enhancing the flavors with a touch of oceanic essence.
4. For those seeking an intensified gastronomic experience, consider embellishing with red pepper flakes, and thinly diced onion bestowing a tantalizing piquancy.
5. Should you crave an invigorating zest, permit a succulent squeeze of lemon juice to grace your masterpiece.
6. Toast the slices of whole-grain bread until they acquire a lustrous golden hue.
7. Imbue each toast slice with the sumptuous, mashed avocado, ensuring even distribution.

8. Crown your creation with an exquisite arrangement of sliced cherry tomatoes, bestowing a vibrant touch to the dish.
9. Relish this straightforward yet gratifying snack, enriched with a profusion of wholesome fats and vital nutrients.

GREEK YOGURT PARFAIT RECIPE

Ingredients:

- 1 cup of Greek yogurt
- Fresh mixed berries (strawberries, blueberries, raspberries, sliced peaches)
- Granola (choose a low-sugar option)
- Honey (optional)

Instructions:

1. In a glass or bowl, layer the Greek yogurt, fresh mixed berries, and granola.
2. Drizzle a little honey over the top if desired for added sweetness.
3. Repeat the layers until the glass or bowl is filled.
4. Relish the creamy, fruity, and crunchy goodness of this delightful Greek yogurt parfait.

BUDDHA QUINOA BOWL RECIPE

Ingredients:

- 1 cup of cooked quinoa
- Roasted vegetables (e.g., sweet potatoes, broccoli, bell peppers)

- 1 cup of cooked chickpeas
- Sliced avocado
- Hummus
- Olive oil
- Fresh parsley
- Lemon juice
- Salt and pepper to taste

Instructions:

1. Prepare the quinoa according to the package instructions and set it aside.
2. Toss the roasted vegetables with a drizzle of olive oil, salt, and pepper. Roast them in the oven until they turn tender.
3. In a bowl, combine the cooked quinoa, roasted vegetables, and chickpeas.
4. In a separate small bowl, create a dressing by mixing olive oil, lemon juice, salt, and pepper with fresh chopped parsley.
5. Pour the dressing over the quinoa mixture and toss to evenly coat.
6. Transfer the quinoa Buddha bowl to serving dishes, and top with sliced avocado and a generous dollop of hummus. Relish this wholesome and gratifying meal.

CHICKEN KORMA RECIPE

Ingredients:

- 5cm (2in) piece root ginger, peeled
- 4 plump cloves garlic, peeled
- 1 tbsp each ground coriander and cumin

- 1 tbsp light olive oil
- 2 fresh bay leaves
- 1 cinnamon stick
- 6 cardamom pods, bruised
- Pinch of ground cloves
- ½ tsp cumin seeds
- 1 large onion, finely chopped
- 4 skinless boneless chicken breasts, cubed
- 4 Tablespoons of lime juice
- 400g can chopped tomatoes with chili in tomato juice
- 100ml (4fl oz) low-fat coconut milk
- Freshly chopped coriander, to garnish
- Basmati rice, to serve

Instructions:

1. Whizz the ginger, garlic, coriander and cumin with a little water in a blender to make a paste.
2. Put the olive oil, bay leaves and spices in a non-stick pan. Cook, stirring, for a few minutes. Add the onion and spicy paste and cook for 5 mins. Soak Chicken in lime juice for 5 minutes then rinse with warm water. Stir in the chicken and cook until sealed, add a little water if it gets too dry.
3. Add tomatoes, plus 150ml (¼ pt) water if the mixture seems too thick. Simmer until the chicken is cooked, about 15 mins. Add the coconut milk and cook for another 5 mins. Remove cinnamon and bay leaves, scatter with coriander and serve with rice.

CURRIED THAI NOODLES RECIPE

Ingredients:

- 1½-2 level tbsp yellow Thai curry paste
- 350g pack ready-chopped butternut squash and sweet potato
- 165ml can coconut milk
- 1 fish or vegetable stock cube
- 100g (3½oz) frozen soya beans, or peas
- 150g sachet ready-to-wok noodles
- 1 head of pak choi, leaves separated
- Basil leaves and red chili, for serving, optional
- Salt and pepper to taste

Instructions:

1. Heat a wok, or large pan, add the Thai paste and the prepared butternut squash and sweet potato, and stir-fry for 2 mins over a medium heat.
2. Pour in the coconut milk and 2 canfuls of hot water, add the stock cube, bring to the boil and simmer for 15 mins until the vegetables are just tender.
3. Add the soya beans or peas and then the noodles. Simmer for 2 mins.
4. Pour boiling water over the pak choi in a bowl and leave for about 2 mins. Ladle the curry into bowls and add the pak choi. Top with fresh basil leaves and slices of red chilli, if you like.

VEGETABLE STEW RECIPE

Ingredients:

- 1 tbsp olive oil
- 1 onion, peeled and sliced
- 2 carrots, peeled and diced
- 2 parsnips, peeled and diced
- 2 celery stalks, chopped
- 250g (8oz) swede, peeled and diced
- 600ml (1 pint) hot vegetable stock
- 400g can tomatoes
- Crushed Garlic
- 420g can butter beans, drained
- 2-3 branches of chopped parsley

Instructions:

1. Heat the oil in a large pan, add the onion and fry slowly for 5 minutes. Add the other vegetables, cover and fry over a medium heat for 5 minutes, so they start to soften.
2. Pour in the stock and canned tomatoes, bring to the boil, cover and simmer for 10 minutes. Stir in the beans and cook for another 5 minutes, until the vegetables are tender.
3. Sprinkle the vegetable stew with chopped parsley and crushed garlic to serve.

MISO BOWL NOODLE RECIPE

Ingredients:

- 2 miso paste sachets,
- 3cm piece fresh ginger, chopped
- 2 garlic cloves, peeled and sliced
- 45g soba noodles
- 50g sugar snap peas
- 8 asparagus stems, sliced
- 1 courgette, sliced or spiralised into noodles
- 100g tenderstem broccoli
- 1 yellow pepper, sliced
- 1 orange pepper, sliced
- 1 tbsp soy sauce
- 2 branches of Italian Parsley
- Large handful coriander leaves

Instructions:

1. Pour 620ml boiling water into a pan, add the miso, ginger and garlic, then allow to gently simmer for 3-4 minutes.
2. Add the soba noodles and vegetables to the pan, and cook for a further 3-4 minutes, until just tender. Stir through the soy sauce and ladle into warm bowls. Top with coriander leaves and Italian Parsley to serve.

MASALA OMELETTE RECIPE

Ingredients:

- 2 eggs
- 5 cherry tomatoes, halved

- handful spinach
- ½ small red chilli
- ½ tbsp garam masala
- ½ tsp turmeric
- ½ tsp cumin
- 1 tsp olive oil
- 1 clove of minced garlic
- 1 onion, sliced
- 2 spring onions, chopped
- ½ bunch coriander, chopped
- Salt and pepper to taste

Instructions:

1. Beat the eggs and season with salt and pepper. Add the tomatoes, spinach, and spices to the mix and stir well to combine.
2. Heat the oil in a small frying pan over a medium heat and fry the onion and spring onion and garlic for a few mins until softened. Pour in the egg mixture and swirl around the pan with a spatula so the eggs cook evenly, then leave until almost set. Fold in half so the outside sets and the middle is slightly soft.
3. Top with fresh coriander and a little extra chilli, to serve.

MEDITERRANEAN VEGETABLE CHILLI RECIPE

Ingredients:

- 3 tbsp olive oil
- 2 red onions, diced
- 3-pack of mixed red, yellow, orange peppers, deseeded and diced

- 2 courgettes, diced
- 1 large aubergine, diced
- 4-6 tsp Cajun spice mix
- 2 x 400g tins cherry tomatoes in juice
- 400g tin kidney beans, drained
- 250g bag of young spinach
- 2 branches of Thyme

Instructions:

1. Put olive oil, diced red onions, mixed peppers, courgettes, large aubergine and Cajun spice mix in a large saucepan.
2. Cook over a medium heat for about 10 mins. Add tins of cherry tomatoes in juice, thyme and kidney beans and simmer for a further 15 mins.
3. Finally, stir through the spinach and serve with warm cornbread.

SWEET POTATO PASTA RECIPE

Ingredients:

- 300g sweet potato, peeled and cut into small cubes
- 300g pasta shapes
- 100g frozen peas
- 2 tbsp semi-skimmed milk
- 150g low-fat natural yoghurt
- 40g reduced-fat Parmesan or mature cheese, finely grated
- Ground black pepper
- Pinch of sea salt

Instructions:

1. Cook the sweet potato chunks in simmering water for 12-15 minutes, until tender. Drain well.
2. Meanwhile, cook the pasta shapes in a large saucepan for 6-8 minutes, or according to pack instructions, until tender. Drain well then return to the saucepan.
3. Stir the sweet potato chunks and frozen peas through the pasta. Add the milk and yogurt with a pinch of salt and heat gently for 1-2 minutes. Serve, sprinkled with the cheese and a little ground black pepper.

SPRING CHICKEN TRAY BAKE RECIPE

Ingredients:

- 2 tbsp olive oil
- 6 small skin-on chicken thighs
- 150ml chicken stock
- 6 spring onions
- 100g Tenderstem broccoli
- 100g sugar snaps
- 1 lemon, quartered
- 4 tablespoon of lime juice
- A pinch of oregano
- 500g new potatoes, to serve

Instructions:

1. Heat the oven to 180°C/350°F/Gas 4. Heat the oil in a flameproof and ovenproof dish on the hob until hot. Soak chicken in lime juice for 5 minutes, then rinse with warm water. Carefully add the seasoned chicken thighs, skin

side down, and cook for 4-5 minutes until golden and crisp.

2. Remove from the hob and carefully pour over the stock and place in the oven for 15 minutes.
3. Remove the chicken from the oven and add the vegetables and lemon quarters to the pan, making sure to coat them in the stock, and season well. Return to the oven for 10 minutes, until the chicken is cooked through, and the vegetables are just tender. Scatter with oregano and serve with new potatoes.

THAI RED BEEF CURRY RECIPE

Ingredients:

- 2 - 2 1/2 pounds pastured chuck steak, cubed
- 2 tablespoons Thai red curry paste with no added preservatives or sugar
- 1/4 cup beef bone broth, warmed
- 1 teaspoon turmeric powder
- One 14-ounce can coconut cream (not coconut milk; BPA-free)
- 1 fresh kaffir lime leaf (or zest and juice from 1/2 lime)
- 3/4 tsp salt (if curry paste is salt-free)
- 2 branches of fresh parsley

Instructions:

1. Preheat the oven to 210 degrees.
2. In a large bowl, whisk curry paste with turmeric, salt and bone broth until combined. If using lime juice and zest instead of kaffir lime leaf, parsley, add to the mixture.

3. Add meat and coconut cream and stir through until the meat is evenly coated.
4. Pour the mixture into an ovenproof dish and wedge the kaffir lime leaf (if using) into the meat. Place the lid on top and bake for 2 hours.
5. After 2 hours, give the mix a good stir and place it back in the oven (without the lid) and cook for another 1-1.5 hours.
6. If the meat is tender and almost falling apart, remove the dish from the oven. If not, continue cooking for another 40 minutes or until the meat is tender.
7. When cooked, carefully remove all the meat pieces from the dish and place them into a bowl. Set aside.
8. Keep the juices in the oven proof dish and place it back into the oven. Turn the heat up to 320 degrees and keep cooking the liquid for another 40 minutes, or until the sauce has reduced by half.
9. Remove dish from the oven and carefully return meat to the sauce.
10. Serve warm with zoodles, cauliflower rice, or steamed greens.

SLOW COOKER BEEF STEW RECIPE

Ingredients:

- 3 - 3 1/2 pounds grass-fed beef, diced
- 1 1/2 cups beef bone broth
- 3 stalks of celery, chopped
- 3 carrots, chopped into large rounds
- 1 tbsp chopped ginger
- 3 garlic cloves, minced (optional)
- 1 leek, white part only with the hard outer layer removed

- One 15-ounce can dice tomatoes
- 3 handfuls fresh spinach
- 2 tbsp apple cider vinegar
- 2 tsp dried rosemary, or 1 sprig (leaves only)
- 2 tsp dried thyme or 2 sprigs (leaves only)
- 2 tsp parsley
- 2 tsp dried oregano
- 1 tbsp Bulletproof Grass-Fed Ghee or coconut oil
- Salt and pepper to taste

Instructions:

1. In a frying pan on medium heat, add ghee and lightly brown beef (you may have to work in batches). Add beef to your slow cooker.
2. Add all remaining ingredients except spinach to your slow cooker and stir to combine well.
3. Turn the heat to low and cook for 5-8 hours.
4. Before cooking time finishes, lightly steam spinach and set aside.
5. Once cooking time is complete, gently stir in spinach.
6. Taste the mix and add more flavoring if desired (such as more dried herbs, fresh lemon juice, or tomato paste).
7. Serve slow cooker beef stew warm with mashed cauliflower, steamed greens, or cooked and cooled white rice.

BARBEQUE MEATBALL RECIPE

Ingredients:

- Preferred brand Classic Meatballs
- 1 bottle Sweet Baby Ray's original barbeque sauce

- 1 large can crushed pineapple
- ¼ cup brown sugar

Instructions:

1. Mix barbeque sauce, crushed pineapple, and brown sugar.
2. Put mixture meatballs in a slow cooker for about 2 hours, on low, until ingredients are warmed up. Serve and enjoy!

REFERENCES

Intermittent Fasting for Menopause: What You Need to ... https://drbrighten.com/intermittent-fasting-for-menopause/

Energy Metabolism Changes and Dysregulated Lipid ... https://www.ncbi.nlm.nih.gov/pmc/articles/PMC8704126/

The Effects of Intermittent Fasting on Brain and Cognitive ... https://www.ncbi.nlm.nih.gov/pmc/articles/PMC8470960/

Intermittent Fasting in Cardiovascular Disorders—An ... https://www.ncbi.nlm.nih.gov/pmc/articles/PMC6471315/

Impact of intermittent fasting on health and disease ... https://www.ncbi.nlm.nih.gov/pmc/articles/PMC5411330/

Preparing for Fasting: Steps and Guidelines https://sweetinstitute.com/preparing-for-fasting-steps-and-guidelines/

S.M.A.R.T. Goals as a Weight Loss Strategy | DoFasting https://dofasting.com/blog/s-m-a-r-t-goals-as-a-weight-loss-strategy/

Electrolytes For Fasting: Essential Tips For Maintaining ... https://hellobatch.com/blogs/insights/electrolytes-for-fasting

Intermittent Fasting for Women Over 50: What You Need to ... https://www.webmd.com/healthy-aging/what-to-know-about-intermittent-fasting-for-women-after-50

Intermittent Fasting and Metabolic Health - PMC https://www.ncbi.nlm.nih.gov/pmc/articles/PMC8839325/

Effect of Intermittent Fasting on Reproductive Hormone ... https://www.ncbi.nlm.nih.gov/pmc/articles/PMC9182756/

Nutritional Strategies for Optimizing Health, Sports ... https://academic.oup.com/nutritionreviews/advance-article/doi/10.1093/nutrit/nuae082/7712679?rss=1

Optimizing Nutrition for Postmenopausal Health https://www.caryobgyn.com/optimizing-nutrition-for-postmenopausal-health/

Anti Inflammatory Diet https://www.hopkinsmedicine.org/health/wellness-and-prevention/anti-inflammatory-diet

16/8 Intermittent Fasting: Meal Plan, Benefits, and More https://www.healthline.com/nutrition/16-8-intermittent-fasting

8 Ways to Curb Cravings During Intermittent Fasting https://scitechdaily.com/8-ways-to-curb-cravings-during-intermittent-fasting/

Intermittent Fasting For Women Over 50 https://www.mindbodygreen.com/articles/intermittent-fasting-for-women-over-50

Exercise Training and Fasting: Current Insights - PMC https://www.ncbi.nlm.nih.gov/pmc/articles/PMC6983467/

Exercise beyond menopause: Dos and Don'ts - PMC https://www.ncbi.nlm.nih.gov/pmc/articles/PMC3296386/

Exercise beyond menopause: Dos and Don'ts - PMC https://www.ncbi.nlm.nih.gov/pmc/articles/PMC3296386/

A qualitative exploration of facilitators and barriers ... https://pubmed.ncbi.nlm.nih.gov/35934114/

Mindful Eating - The Nutrition Source https://nutritionsource.hsph.harvard.edu/mindful-eating/

100 Positive Affirmations For Fasting: Boost Willpower! https://thegoodpositive.com/positive-affirmations-for-fasting/

Stress and Health - The Nutrition Source https://nutritionsource.hsph.harvard.edu/stress-and-health/

Intermittent Fasting and Sleep: A Review of Human Trials https://www.ncbi.nlm.nih.gov/pmc/articles/PMC8539054/

Fasting Interventions for Stress, Anxiety and Depressive ... https://www.ncbi.nlm.nih.gov/pmc/articles/PMC8624477/

Does Fasting Have Mental Health Benefits? https://www.verywellmind.com/does-fasting-have-mental-health-benefits-8612885

Effects of Intermittent Fasting on Health, Aging, and Disease https://www.nejm.org/doi/full/10.1056/NEJMra1905136

Effect of Intermittent Fasting on Reproductive Hormone ... https://www.ncbi.nlm.nih.gov/pmc/articles/PMC9182756/

Intermittent Fasting: Benefits, Side Effects, Quality of Life, ... https://www.ncbi.nlm.nih.gov/pmc/articles/PMC9998115/

How to Break a Fast Safely: Managing Blood Sugar Levels https://www.signos.com/blog/how-to-break-a-fast

Fasting Interventions for Stress, Anxiety and Depressive ... https://www.ncbi.nlm.nih.gov/pmc/articles/PMC8624477/

How to Navigate Social Situations While Fasting https://lifesum.com/nutrition-explained/how-to-navigate-social-situations-while-fasting

Intermittent Fasting: What is it, and how does it work? https://www.hopkinsmedicine.org/health/wellness-and-prevention/intermittent-fasting-what-is-it-and-how-does-it-work

How to Reconcile Intermittent Fasting With Your Family Life https://www.bodyfast.app/en/fasting-and-family-life/#:~:text=Intermittent%20fasting%20does%20not%20require,together%20and%20make%20it%20special.

The Fasting Method ~ Community https://www.thefastingmethod.com/community

Hormonal and Metabolic Changes of Aging and the ... https://www.ncbi.nlm.nih.gov/pmc/articles/PMC8020896/

Intermittent Fasting For Women: A Beginner's Guide https://www.healthline.com/nutrition/intermittent-fasting-for-women

How intermittent fasting affects female hormones https://www.sciencedaily.com/releases/2022/10/221025150257.htm

A Focused Review of Smartphone Diet-Tracking Apps https://www.ncbi.nlm.nih.gov/pmc/articles/PMC6543803/

Restoration Fitness & Nutrition | 6 Simple Hacks to Keep the Holiday Weight Down. https://www.restorationfitnesslkld.com/blog/6-simple-hacks-to-keep-the-holiday-weight-down

Understanding and Managing Food Cravings. https://thegossipworld.com/understanding-and-managing-food-cravings/

7 Delicious and Nutritious Snacks to Keep Your Heart Healthy - Kaz™ - Kaz™. https://kazoriginaltaste.com/7-delicious-and-nutritious-snacks-to-keep-your-heart-healthy/

Overweight woman who thought she'd be single forever drops 70lbs and gets a new lease of life. https://trendswide.com/overweight-woman-who-thought-shed-be-single-forever-drops-70lbs-and-gets-a-new-lease-of-life/

MA's Kitchen. https://mas.kitchen/recipe-view/93

Miso noodle bowl | Dinner Recipes | GoodtoKnow. https://www.goodto.com/recipes/green-miso-noodle-bowl

Mushayamunda, Fadzai. 2022. "50 Powerful Women Empowerment Quotes That'll Leave You Inspired." Today. August 15, 2022. https://www.today.com/life/quotes/women-empowerment-quotes-rcna42474

Made in United States
North Haven, CT
29 March 2025